Math

for Pharmacy
Technicians

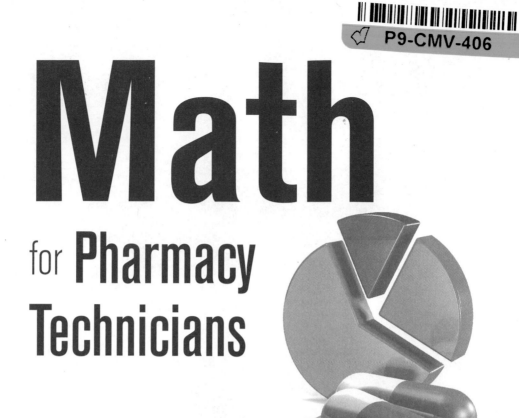

Math

for Pharmacy
Technicians

Lorraine C. Zentz, CPhT, PhD
Pharmacy Technician Program
ed2go/ GES

JONES AND BARTLETT PUBLISHERS

Sudbury, Massachusetts

BOSTON   TORONTO   LONDON   SINGAPORE

World Headquarters
Jones and Bartlett Publishers
40 Tall Pine Drive
Sudbury, MA 01776
978-443-5000
info@jbpub.com
www.jbpub.com

Jones and Bartlett Publishers
Canada
6339 Ormindale Way
Mississauga, Ontario L5V 1J2
Canada

Jones and Bartlett Publishers
International
Barb House, Barb Mews
London W6 7PA
United Kingdom

Jones and Bartlett's books and products are available through most bookstores and online booksellers. To contact Jones and Bartlett Publishers directly, call 800-832-0034, fax 978-443-8000, or visit our website, www.jbpub.com.

Substantial discounts on bulk quantities of Jones and Bartlett's publications are available to corporations, professional associations, and other qualified organizations. For details and specific discount information, contact the special sales department at Jones and Bartlett via the above contact information or send an email to specialsales@jbpub.com.

The author, editor, and publisher have made every effort to provide accurate information. However, they are not responsible for errors, omissions, or for any outcomes related to the use of the contents of this book and take no responsibility for the use of the products and procedures described. Treatments and side effects described in this book may not be applicable to all people; likewise, some people may require a dose or experience a side effect that is not described herein. Drugs and medical devices are discussed that may have limited availability controlled by the Food and Drug Administration (FDA) for use only in a research study or clinical trial. Research, clinical practice, and government regulations often change the accepted standard in this field. When consideration is being given to use of any drug in the clinical setting, the health care provider or reader is responsible for determining FDA status of the drug, reading the package insert, and reviewing prescribing information for the most up-to-date recommendations on dose, precautions, and contraindications, and determining the appropriate usage for the product. This is especially important in the case of drugs that are new or seldom used.

Production Credits
Publisher: David Cella
Associate Editor: Maro Gartside
Editorial Assistant: Teresa Reilly
Production Manager: Julie Champagne Bolduc
Production Assistant: Jessica Steele Newfell
Marketing Manager: Grace Richards
Manufacturing and Inventory Control Supervisor: Amy Bacus
Composition: International Typesetting and Composition
Cover Design: Scott Moden
Cover and Title Page Image: © Norebbo/Dreamstime.com
Printing and Binding: Malloy, Inc.
Cover Printing: John Pow Company

Library of Congress Cataloging-in-Publication Data
Zentz, Lorraine C.
  Math for pharmacy technicians / Lorraine C. Zentz.
     p. ; cm.
  Includes index.
  ISBN 978-0-7637-5961-2 (pbk. : alk. paper)
  1. Pharmaceutical arithmetic. 2. Pharmacy technicians. I. Title.
  [DNLM: 1. Drug Dosage Calculations. 2. Mathematics. 3. Pharmaceutical Preparations—
administration & dosage. QV 748 Z56m 2010]
  RS57.Z46 2010
  615'.1401513—dc22
                                    2009025969
6048
Printed in the United States of America
13 12 11 10 09   10 9 8 7 6 5 4 3 2 1

Contents

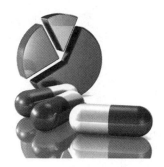

Introduction

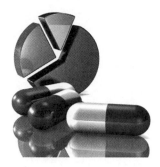

An essential tool for all pharmacy technicians is a full grasp of the necessary math skills needed on a daily basis in the pharmacy setting. Simply understanding the math is not enough: technicians must have the confidence to arrive at an accurate answer. While drugs can be of great help to patients, they also are powerful and potentially deadly chemicals that must be treated with the utmost respect; proper dosing is critical. Misplaced decimals, extra zeros, or "close enough" measuring are unacceptable.

Utilizing a straightforward layout, *Math for Pharmacy Technicians* focuses on the crucial terminology (terms and abbreviations) pertaining to calculating medication dosages. This text provides more than just the final answer: easy-to-follow explanations show how to complete math equations and conversions and boxed text (featuring tips, key points, and reminders) help students comprehend the material in a manner that will be beneficial when solving future problems both in this book and on the job.

The basic math skills a pharmacy technician is required to understand include fractions, decimals, and percentages. In *Math for Pharmacy Technicians*, different methods are demonstrated so that technicians will feel confident in the skills they are learning. There may be several ways to reach a solution, but technicians must understand the quickest and most accurate way to reach a solution. Practice, such as focusing on the Practice Problems and Chapter Quizzes available in this text, will help to determine the method appropriate for each situation. After completing the examples and checking the answers against the Answer Key (see Appendix A), technicians will be ready to tackle math in the pharmacy setting.

Fundamentals of Math

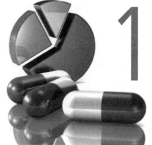

OBJECTIVES

- Understand the difference between the Arabic and Roman numeral systems
- Translate Arabic numerals to Roman numerals
- Translate Roman numerals to Arabic numerals
- Understand the metric system
- Understand the apothecary system
- Be able to convert metric to apothecary
- Be able to convert apothecary to metric

ARABIC NUMERALS

The Arabic number system uses the numerals 1, 2, 3, 4, 5, 6, 7, 8, 9, and zero (0). It is also known as the decimal system. Depending on how these numbers are arranged determines the value of the number. For example, digits 4, 7, and 2 placed together (472) represent the number four hundred seventy-two.

A decimal point (.) separates whole numbers, or units, from fractional numbers, or fractional units. All numbers on the left side of the decimal point are considered whole numbers. All numbers placed on the right of the decimal point are considered fractional units, or less than one whole unit. The following number line shows the relationship of Arabic numerals based on their position in a number.

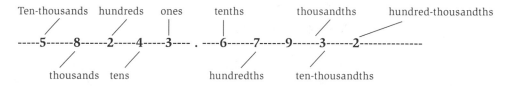

The number 43.6 contains the numerals 4, 3, and 6. This represents forty-three units of one and six-tenths of one unit. Decimals will be covered in more detail in Chapter 2.

ROMAN NUMERALS

Remember:
Dates are always
capital letters
MCMXC (1990).

The Roman numeral system does not utilize numerals. Instead, the putting together of alpha characters that follow specific rules represent each number. The alpha characters used are **c, d, i, l, m, s, v,** and **x.** These letters can be small case or capitalized—it does not matter. One exception is that dates (2009) always use capital letters. Each letter represents a specific number.

ss = $\frac{1}{2}$

I or i = 1

V or v = 5

X or x = 10

L or l = 50

C or c = 100

D or d = 500

M or m = 1000

The Roman numeral system is not used to do calculations. It is used to document values or quantities only. In order to perform calculations, Roman numerals have to be converted to Arabic numerals. Once you know the rules, this becomes easy to do. When a number is represented by two letters, and the second letter corresponds to a number with the same value or a smaller value than the first one, you add them together.

VI = 5 + 1 = 6

II = 1 + 1 = 2

XV = 10 + 5 = 15

When there are two letters and the second one represents a number with a greater value than the first letter, you subtract the first from the second.

IX = I → 1, X → 10, 10 – 1 = 9

XL = X → 10, L → 50, 50 – 10 = 40

When there are more than two letters used to represent a number, you apply the subtraction rule first. Remember, you subtract any smaller value letter from a larger value letter that follows it. Once that is done, you add all the values together to determine the number.

XLIV = X → 10, L → 50, 50 – 10 = 40; I → 1, V → 5, 5 – 1 = 4; 40 + 4 = 44

CXXIV = C → 100, X → 10, I → 1, V → 5; 100 + 10 + 10 + (5 – 1) = 124

CCXLIX = 100 + 100 + (50 – 10) + (10 – 1) = 249

Practice Problems 1.1

Convert the Arabic to the Roman.

1. 2010 _____
2. 1949 _____
3. 24 _____
4. 520 _____
5. 13 _____

6. 93 _____
7. 42 _____
8. 375 _____
9. 6 _____
10. 787 _____

11. 400 _____
12. 231 _____
13. 86 _____
14. 66 _____
15. 39 _____

16. 161 _____   20. 999 _____   24. 77 _____
17. 684 _____   21. 315 _____   25. 104 _____
18. 57 _____   22. 18 _____
19. 1496 _____   23. 540 _____

Convert the Roman to the Arabic.

26. MMVII _____   35. dc _____   44. CCL _____
27. dxxiv _____   36. MCDLVI _____   45. mv _____
28. cix _____   37. vi _____   46. XXI _____
29. LIII _____   38. xxxvi _____   47. xliii _____
30. XLIX _____   39. iii _____   48. MCMLXXXII _____
31. iv _____   40. LXXV _____   49. xxviii _____
32. viii _____   41. ccxxiv _____   50. MDCCXCVI _____
33. CCCXXIV _____ 42. mmmcccxxix _____
34. LXI _____   43. dxliv _____

METRIC SYSTEM

The measurement systems in place for pharmacy are:

- Metric
- Avoirdupois
- Apothecary

The avoirdupois system is based on British standards and states that 1 pound is equivalent to 16 ounces. Apothecary systems used the base of grains and minims. They are still seen in pharmacy calculations today. Other units you will see in the apothecary system are drams, ounces, and pounds.

The most common system is metric. The three basic units of measure are meter, gram, and liter. The two most common units in pharmacy are grams (weight) and liters (volume). The liter is based on the volume of 1000 cubic centimeters (cc) of water. One cubic centimeter is equivalent to 1 milliliter (ml), so 1000 mL equals 1 liter. The gram is based on the weight of 1 cubic centimeter of distilled water at 4°C.

The metric system was developed in the late 18th century in France. The United States adopted this system in the late 1800s and made it our standard of measure in 1893. It is the accepted system of measure for scientists all around the world because of its simplicity.

The liter is the base unit for measuring liquid volumes in the metric system. It represents the volume of a cube that is one-tenth of a meter on each side. The most common units used for volume in pharmacy are the liter, milliliter, and microliter. **Table 1.1** displays the measures of metric volume.

Use the liter as your homebase. Kilo- and milli- represent 1000. Multiplying by 1000 will get you to kilo- (small to large) and dividing by 1000 will get you to milli- (large to small). Hecto- and centi- represent 100. Deka- and deci- represent 10.

When doing calculations with metric measures, you must be sure all your values are in the same measure. If your final answer needs to be in milligrams (mg)

Remember:
It takes lots of small parts to equal one large part!

Remember:
It only takes a portion of a large part to equal a smaller part.

TABLE 1.1   **Metric Volumes**

Volume Label	Abbreviation	Liters	Comparison to a Liter
Kiloliter	kL	1000	0.001 kL
Hectoliter	hL	100	0.01 hL
Dekaliter	dkL	10	0.1 dkL
Liter	L	1	1.0 L
Deciliter	dL	0.1	10 dL
Centiliter	cL	0.01	100 cL
Milliliter	mL	0.001	1000 mL
Microliter	mcL (μL)	0.000001	1,000,000 mcL

and you are dealing with grams (g), you need to convert your values into the desired measure. You can do this before you begin, or once the calculations are completed. If you are dealing with multiple measures, you need to convert them all into one common measure. To convert from a large measure to a smaller one, you need to multiply. To convert from small measures to large measures, division is the tool to use.

■ EXAMPLE 1

You have a 3 L bottle of cough syrup. How many milliliters are in this container?

3 L
(1 L = 1000 mL)
3 L × 1000 = 3000 mL

■ EXAMPLE 2

You have an IV bag that contains 600 mL. How many liters is this?

1. 1 L
   (1 L = 1000 mL)
   1 × 1000 mL = 1000 mL
2. 600 mL ÷ 1000 mL = 0.6 L
   (1000 mL = 1 L)

■ EXAMPLE 3

A 5 L bag of fluid contains how many microliters?

1. 5 L
   (1 L = 1000 mL)
   5 × 1000 mL = 5000 mL (milliliters)
2. 5000 mL
   (1 mL = 1000 mcL)
   5000 × 1000 = 5,000,000 mcL (microliters)

Practice Problems 1.2

Convert the following.

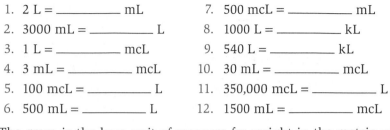

1. 2 L = _____ mL
2. 3000 mL = _____ L
3. 1 L = _____ mcL
4. 3 mL = _____ mcL
5. 100 mcL = _____ L
6. 500 mL = _____ L

7. 500 mcL = _____ mL
8. 1000 L = _____ kL
9. 540 L = _____ kL
10. 30 mL = _____ mcL
11. 350,000 mcL = _____ L
12. 1500 mL = _____ mcL

The gram is the base unit of measure for weight in the metric system. It represents the weight of 1 cubic meter (cm^3) of water at 4°C. The amount, or concentration, of a drug is measured in metric weight. The most common measures used are grams, milligrams, and micrograms. A person's weight is also converted to kilograms, from pounds, in order to calculate the dose of medication necessary for treatment. **Table 1.2** displays the measures of metric weight.

The most common conversions are micrograms → milligrams, milligrams → grams, and grams → kilograms.

1000 mcg = 1 mg
1000 mg = 1 g
1000 g = 1 kg

■ **EXAMPLE 4**

How many mg are in 5.4 g?

(1 g = 1000 mg)
5.4 × 1000 = 5400 mg

Remember that you want to know how many small parts are in the big part.

■ **EXAMPLE 5**

Convert 15,000 mg to grams.

15,000 ÷ 1000 = 15 g

TABLE 1.2   **Metric Weights**

Weight Label	Abbreviation	Grams	Comparison to a Gram
Kilogram	kg	1000	0.001 kg
Hectogram	hg	100	0.01 hg
Dekagram	dkg	10	0.1 dkg
Gram	g	1	1 g
Decigram	dg	0.1	10 dg
Centigram	cg	0.01	100 cg
Milligram	mg	0.001	1000 mg
Microgram	mcg (μg)	0.000001	1,000,000 mcg

▪ **EXAMPLE 6**

150,000 mcg is equivalent to how many grams?

(1 g = 1000 mg)
(1 mg = 1000 mcg)
150,000 ÷ 1000 = 150 mg ÷ 1000 = 0.15 g

Practice Problems 1.3

Convert the following.

1. 2 g = _____ mcg
2. 1 mg = _____ mcg
3. 100 mg = _____ g
4. 2 kg = _____ g
5. 5 kg = _____ mg
6. 4000 mcg = _____ mg
7. 3 g = _____ mg
8. 500 mg = _____ g
9. 630 mg = _____ kg
10. 5.4 kg = _____ g
11. 0.2 mg = _____ mcg
12. 4 g = _____ kg
13. 250 mcg = _____ mg
14. 0.5 mg = _____ mcg
15. 22 g = _____ mg
16. 320 mcg = _____ g

Metric Conversions

Converting different measurements to a common one makes it easier to perform calculations. There are many different types of measurements. The most common used by people outside the medical and scientific community are the household measurements (e.g., tsp, tbsp, ounce, quart, gallon). While these are the least accurate, they are the easiest ones to direct patients on dosing at home. The common tablespoon can vary from 15 mL up to 22 mL in measurement. The accurate dose of a tablespoon is 15 mL when comparing to the metric system. Knowing common conversions can help ensure that proper doses are being calculated and dispensed. Most retail pharmacies will send a dispensing spoon home with liquid medications because it has "mL" markings along with teaspoon/tablespoon markings to ensure accurate dosing.

▪ **EXAMPLE 7**

A medication has 5 mg/mL and the patient needs to take 1 tablespoon four times a day.

If the patient takes 15 mL per dose, he or she would receive 60 mL daily. If he or she took 22 mL per dose, that would be 88 mL daily. At 60 mL daily, the patient receives 300 mg (prescribed). At 88 mL daily, the patient receives 440 mg (overdose).

Conversions are done in relation to the metric system. The metric system is always used to perform calculations. **Table 1.3** lists some common conversions that should be committed to memory. These are used almost daily in the pharmacy. Many products list both measures on their labels. The United States may be the only country in the world that does not use the metric system as their standard.

Practice this exercise to become familiar with common conversions:

1 tsp = 5 mL
1 tbsp = 3 tsp = 15 mL
2 tbsp = 6 tsp = 30 mL = 1 ounce

TABLE 1.3 **Household to Metric Conversions**

Household Measure	Metric Measure
1 teaspoon	5 mL
1 tablespoon	15 mL
1 ounce	30 mL
8 ounces ($\frac{1}{2}$ pint)	240 mL
1 pint (16 ounces)	473 mL (480 mL)
1 quart (32 ounces)	946 mL
1 gallon (128 ounces)	3785 mL
1 pound (lb)	454 g
2.2 pounds (lbs)	1 kg

Practice Problems 1.4

Convert the following.

1. $\frac{1}{2}$ tsp = _____ mL   a. 1.55   b. 2.5   c. 1.75
2. 3 tsp = _____ mL   a. 10   b. 12   c. 15
3. 2 pints = _____ mL   a. 946   b. 900   c. 500
4. $\frac{1}{2}$ lb = _____ g   a. 225   b. 227   c. 300
5. 3 qts = _____ mL   a. 2838   b. 2800   c. 3000
6. 3 tbsp = _____ mL   a. 40   b. 48   c. 45
7. 2 oz = _____ mL   a. 60   b. 65   c. 75
8. 3 oz = _____ mL   a. 80   b. 90   c. 95
9. 45 mL = _____ oz   a. 1.5   b. 2   c. 3
10. 15 mL = _____ tsp   a. 2   b. 3   c. 4
11. $\frac{1}{4}$ tsp = _____ mL   a. $\frac{1}{2}$ b. $\frac{1}{4}$ c. 1.25
12. 20 mL = _____ tsp   a. 4   b. 5   c. 6
13. 100 kg = _____ lbs   a. 120   b. 100   c. 220
14. 66 lbs = _____ kg   a. 33   b. 30   c. 20
15. 1892 mL = _____ gal   a. $\frac{1}{2}$ b. $\frac{3}{4}$ c. 1
16. 2 qts = _____ pts   a. 2   b. 4   c. 3
17. 8 oz = _____ tsp   a. 48   b. 24   c. 12
18. 7.5 mL = _____ tsp   a. 3   b. $1\frac{1}{2}$ c. $\frac{1}{2}$
19. 45 mL = _____ tbsp   a. 3   b. 2   c. 1
20. 8 oz = _____ tbsp   a. 8   b. 6   c. 16

APOTHECARY SYSTEM

The apothecary system uses the measure units of minims, drams, and grains for smaller measures, and then progresses to ounces, pints, quarts, gallons, and pounds as seen in the household measure system. This system is seldom used

TABLE 1.4   **Apothecary Conversions**

Apothecary	Abbreviation/Symbol	Household Conversion	Metric Conversion
1 minim	ℳ		0.06 mL
16.23 minims	ℳ		1 mL
1 dram	℥	1 teaspoon (5 mL)	3.69 mL (4 mL)
8 drams (volume)	℥	1 ounce (6 drams)	29.57 mL (30 mL)
8 drams (weight)	℥	1 ounce	30 g
1 grain	gr		65 mg
15.4 grains	gr		1 g
1 pound	lb	1 pound	454 g

For calculating purposes, 6 drams = 1 oz based on the dram being 5 mL, even though the true measure would be 8 drams (4 mL).

anymore but does make an appearance in pharmacy occasionally. For calculation purposes, these units are also converted to metric. (See **Table 1.4**.)

The liquid measures are minims, drams, ounces, pints, quarts, and gallons. You will occasionally see prescriptions written with drams as a unit of measure and, very rarely, the unit of minims is used. A dram is a little less than a teaspoon. Typically, it is converted to a teaspoon measure (5 mL) when calculating or dispensing liquid medications.

The weight measure of grains is still used today for many medications (e.g., aspirin, 5 grains). Many older medications are still measured in grains also (e.g., thyroid, phenobarbital). You will often see both grains and milligrams on the packaging of medications that are dispensed with grains as their unit of measure. Some examples would be aspirin 5 grains (325 mg) tablets or phenobarbital 1 grain (65 mg) tablets.

Grains
Sometimes
1 gr = 60 mg.

It depends
on the
manufacturer:
Codeine
1 gr = 60 mg
Phenobarb
1 gr = 65 mg

Practice Problems 1.5

Convert the following.

		a.	b.	c.
1.	3 gr = _____ mg	a. 185	b. 190	c. 195
2.	$\frac{1}{2}$ gr = _____ mg	a. 32	b. 32.5	c. 33
3.	4 drams = _____ oz	a. $\frac{1}{2}$	b. 1	c. 3
4.	130 mg = _____ gr	a. 2	b. 3	c. 4
5.	2 oz = _____ g	a. 30	b. 45	c. 60
6.	30 mL = _____ drams	a. 8	b. 6	c. 3
7.	4 oz = _____ g	a. 100	b. 120	c. 140
8.	$\frac{1}{2}$ dram = _____ tsp	a. 2	b. $\frac{1}{2}$	c. 3

CHAPTER 1 QUIZ

Convert the following Arabic numerals to Roman numerals.

1. 84
2. 310
3. 490
4. 19
5. 28

Convert the following Roman numerals to Arabic numerals.

1. MCMXCVI
2. CCXXXIV
3. XCV
4. MMIX
5. DCCC

Perform the following conversions.

1. 3 L = _____ mL
2. 2 g = _____ mcg
3. 500 mL = _____ L
4. 3 kg = _____ mg
5. 5000 mcL = _____ L
6. 700 mg = _____ mcg
7. 1.5 L = _____ mL
8. 650 mcg = _____ mg
9. 100 mL = _____ mcL
10. 3500 g = _____ kg
11. 2 L = _____ mcL
12. 4.5 g = _____ mg
13. 300 mL _____ mcL
14. 5 kg = _____ g
15. 8,000 mcL = _____ mL
16. 450 mg = _____ g
17. 1300 mL = _____ L
18. 6 g = _____ mcg
19. 4.2 L = _____ mL
20. 8200 mg = _____ g

Convert the following household measures.

1. 2 tsp = _____ mL
2. 2 pts = _____ mL
3. 2 lbs = _____ g
4. 2 qts = _____ mL

5. 3 tbsp = _____ mL

6. 176 lbs = _____ kg

7. 6 oz = _____ tsp

8. 5 gr = _____ mg

9. 5 oz = _____ g

10. 650 mg = _____ gr

11. 8 oz = _____ mL

12. 25 kg = _____ lbs

13. 15 mL = _____ tsp

14. 60 mL = _____ tbsp

15. 120 mL = _____ oz

16. 180 g = _____ oz

17. 7.5 mL = _____ tsp

18. $\frac{1}{4}$ tsp = _____ mL

19. 45 mL = _____ tbsp

20. 275 lbs = _____ kg

Fractions and Decimals

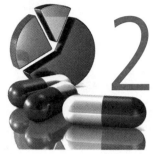

C H A P T E R

2

OBJECTIVES

- Be able to interpret fractions
- Be able to interpret decimals
- Be able to add and subtract fractions
- Be able to add and subtract decimals
- Be able to multiply and divide fractions
- Be able to multiply and divide decimals
- Determine the significant figures for decimals

FRACTIONS

A fraction represents a portion of a whole unit. Numerically, it is expressed as one number over another ($\frac{2}{6}$). The bottom number defines the number of parts it will take to make the whole unit. The top number defines how many parts of the whole there are. (See **Figure 2.1**.)

A fraction is made up of two components: the **numerator** and the **denominator**.

$\underline{2}$ → numerator
6 → denominator

The numerator defines the number of units in the whole you have or need. The denominator represents how many units make up the whole.

A fraction that has the same number in the numerator and the denominator equals one whole; meaning the number of units you have makes the whole complete. If you have eight pieces of pie and the pie pan holds eight pieces, then you have the whole pie.

A. $\dfrac{6}{6} = 1$ **B.** $\dfrac{7}{7} = 1$ **C.** $\dfrac{10}{10} = 1$

You can verify this by dividing the top number by the bottom number ($6 \div 6 = 1$). A number divided by itself is always one.

FIGURE 2.1   Fractions

Whole = $\frac{6}{6}$ or 1   2 units = $\frac{2}{6}$ of the whole

A **proper fraction** is one that has a smaller number on top (numerator). This represents a number that is less than one.

A. $\frac{1}{3}$ **B.** $\frac{3}{7}$ **C.** $\frac{5}{6}$ **D.** $\frac{9}{12}$

When you divide the top number by the bottom number, you get a number less than one.

A. $1 \div 3 = 0.33$ **B.** $3 \div 7 = 0.43$ **C.** $5 \div 6 = 0.83$ **D.** $9 \div 12 = 0.75$

An **improper fraction** is a fraction that has a larger number on top (numerator). This number would represent a whole plus a portion of another whole.

A. $\frac{5}{4} = (1)\frac{4}{4} + \frac{1}{4}$ **B.** $\frac{8}{5} = (1)\frac{5}{5} + \frac{3}{5}$ **C.** $\frac{9}{7} = (1)\frac{7}{7} + \frac{2}{7}$

When you divide the top number by the bottom number, you get a whole plus a number less than one.

A. $5 \div 4 = 1.25$ or $1\frac{1}{4}$ **B.** $8 \div 5 = 1.6$ or $1\frac{3}{5}$ **C.** $9 \div 7 = 1.29$ or $1\frac{2}{7}$

A **mixed number** is a whole number with a fraction. You must make this number into an improper fraction in order to perform any calculations. To do this, you would multiply the bottom number in the fraction by the whole number, add the top number to that product, and then place that value in the numerator position over the original denominator.

$$4\frac{3}{5} = 4 \times 5 = 20 + 3 = 23 \rightarrow \frac{23}{5}$$

A **complex fraction** is a value that has a fraction in both the numerator and denominator position.

$$\frac{\frac{1}{3}}{\frac{5}{8}}$$

Addition and Subtraction

Adding and subtracting fractions requires a few rules in order to obtain the correct answer. When you add or subtract fractions, they must have the same denominator, or **common denominator**. Comparing "apples to apples" is another way to look at it. If you want to know how many apples you have, you can only add or subtract the apples. If you include the oranges, you will not get the correct answer.

To find a common denominator, you need to determine a number that both denominators have in common (common denominator). It could be one of the numbers in the fractions, or you may have to find a different number that is common to both.

■ EXAMPLE 1

$$\frac{3}{12} + \frac{7}{12} = \frac{10}{12} \qquad \frac{11}{12} - \frac{4}{12} = \frac{7}{12}$$

The denominators are the same (12), so you can just add or subtract the numerators and place them over the existing denominator.

■ EXAMPLE 2

$$\frac{2}{3} + \frac{1}{9} =$$

The denominators are different (apples/oranges) so a common factor must be found.

Looking at these two numbers, we see that the 3 will go into the 9 (3 is a factor of 9). We need to rewrite the equation using 9 as the denominator for both fractions. You need to determine what must be done with the 3 in the first fraction to get it to equal 9. Whatever you do to the 3 (denominator), you must also do to the 2 (numerator) in order to keep the fraction equivalent.

$$\frac{2}{3} \times \frac{3}{3} = \frac{6}{9}$$

Now your equation looks like this:

$$\frac{6}{9} + \frac{1}{9} = \frac{7}{9}$$

When it is not so obvious what the common denominator is, you need to follow a different strategy.

■ EXAMPLE 3

$$\frac{2}{15} + \frac{5}{6}$$

You need to list multiples of each denominator to see if they have one in common.

15 = 15, **30**, 45, 60, 75
 6 = 6, 12, 18, 24, **30**, 36, 42

The list shows that 30 is the first multiple that they share. The next step is to create your new equivalent fractions.

$$\frac{2}{15} \times \frac{2}{2} = \frac{4}{30} \qquad \text{and} \qquad \frac{5}{6} \times \frac{5}{5} = \frac{25}{30}$$

Your new equation looks like this: $\frac{4}{30} + \frac{25}{30} = \frac{29}{30}$

Sometimes the only way to find a common denominator is to multiply them together because their product *is* the only thing common.

■ EXAMPLE 4

$$\frac{5}{9} - \frac{3}{7}$$

Looking at these numbers you might assume that they do not have a common multiple other than their product (multiplying them).

Their common denominator is $7 \times 9 = \mathbf{63}$.

$$\frac{5}{9} \times \frac{7}{7} = \frac{35}{63} \qquad \text{and} \qquad \frac{3}{7} \times \frac{9}{9} = \frac{27}{63}$$

Your new equation is

$$\frac{35}{63} - \frac{27}{63} = \frac{8}{63}$$

If your equation has a mixed fraction, be sure to make it into an improper fraction, and then follow these steps to ensure common denominators are present.

Practice Problems 2.1

Simplify the answer to a proper fraction in its simplest terms.

1. $\frac{4}{5} + \frac{4}{5} =$

2. $\frac{3}{8} + \frac{2}{8} =$

3. $\frac{5}{12} + \frac{6}{24} =$

4. $\frac{1}{3} + \frac{4}{9} =$

5. $\frac{8}{27} + \frac{7}{8} =$

6. $\frac{9}{7} + \frac{2}{7} =$

7. $\frac{6}{7} - \frac{2}{7} =$

8. $\frac{7}{9} - \frac{1}{3} =$

9. $\frac{7}{15} + \frac{4}{60} =$

10. $\frac{3}{13} + \frac{4}{7} =$

11. $4\frac{3}{4} + \frac{7}{4} =$

12. $\frac{8}{5} + 2\frac{1}{10} =$

13. $5\frac{2}{3} - 2\frac{1}{3} =$

14. $\frac{12}{7} + \frac{3}{7} =$

15. $\frac{6}{21} + \frac{4}{21} =$

Multiplication and Division

Multiplying fractions is one of the simpler calculations to perform. You do not need to worry about common denominators. The numerators are multiplied together and then the denominators are multiplied together. The answer is then simplified to its lowest term.

■ EXAMPLE 5

$$\frac{3}{8} \times \frac{4}{6} = \frac{3 \times 4}{8 \times 6} = \frac{12}{48} \div \frac{12}{12} = \frac{1}{4}$$

Multiplying the numerators you get 12 and then multiplying the denominators equals 48. The fraction $\frac{12}{48}$ can be simplified to $\frac{1}{4}$ because 12 is a common factor in both the numerator and the denominator.

■ EXAMPLE 6

$$\frac{4}{6} \times \frac{2}{7} \times \frac{3}{5} = \frac{4 \times 2 \times 3}{6 \times 7 \times 5} = \frac{24}{210} \div \frac{2}{2} = \frac{12}{105}$$

Dividing fractions is done using multiplication also. When you divide two fractions, you will invert, or use the reciprocal, of the second fraction and then perform multiplication to solve the equation.

■ EXAMPLE 7

$$\frac{6}{11} \div \frac{3}{8} = \frac{6 \times 8}{11 \times 3} = \frac{48}{33} = 1\frac{15}{33} = 1\frac{5}{11}$$

Solving this equation requires you to "flip" the second fraction and then multiply the numerators together followed by multiplying the denominators together. Simplifying the answer to its lowest terms makes it easier to read and determine its true value.

This answer is in the form of an improper fraction (the numerator is larger than the denominator). To make this a proper or mixed fraction, you need to pull out the "whole" number (1) and determine the remaining fraction. The "one" would be $\frac{33}{33}$. This leaves a remainder of 15 (48 − 33). Following the above equation, the 15 is then placed over the 33 once again. Looking at this fraction $\frac{15}{33}$, you notice that both numbers have a three (3) in common. Simplifying this to its lowest form means dividing both the numerator and the denominator by the common factor (3) to result in a fraction of $\frac{5}{11}$.

■ EXAMPLE 8

$$\frac{8}{3/5} = \frac{8}{1} \times \frac{5}{3} = \frac{40}{3} = 13\frac{1}{3}$$

Remember:
A fraction is simply another way to write a division problem!

The same process is used if there is a fraction in the denominator of a fraction. Simply bring it out of the denominator position and invert it. Follow the multiplication process and reduce to lowest terms if necessary.

Practice Problems 2.2

Solve the following equations and simplify.

1. $\frac{5}{7} \times \frac{4}{8} =$

2. $\frac{2}{4} \times \frac{8}{13} =$

3. $\frac{12}{13} \times \frac{3}{5} =$

4. $\frac{3}{7} \times \frac{2}{9} \times \frac{1}{4} =$

5. $\frac{1}{4} \times \frac{2}{3} \times \frac{5}{6} =$

6. $2\frac{3}{4} \times \frac{7}{8} \times 1\frac{1}{4} =$

7. $\frac{11}{12} \div \frac{3}{4} =$

8. $\frac{5}{6} \div \frac{1}{3} =$

9. $9 \div \frac{4}{5} =$

10. $\frac{1}{5} \div 6 =$

11. $3\frac{1}{2} \div \frac{7}{8} =$

12. $2\frac{3}{4} \div 1\frac{5}{8} =$

DECIMALS

A decimal is another way to represent fractional parts of a whole unit. To convert a fraction to a decimal, you simply divide the numerator by the denominator.

■ **EXAMPLE 9**

$$\frac{3}{4} = 3 \div 4 = 0.75$$

Positionally, each digit to the right or the left of the decimal represents a fractional multiple of 10. The most common fractional units (right of the decimal) seen in pharmacy math are tenths (0.1), hundredths (0.01), and thousandths (0.001).

Many drugs are dosed in fractional units—less than one. When this occurs, it is important to utilize a leading zero in front of the decimal so that no mistake is made in interpreting the desired dose.

■ **EXAMPLE 10**

Levothyroxine 0.15 mg versus .15 mg

Digoxin 0.125 mg versus .125 mg

The levothyroxine could be misinterpreted as 15 mg if you could not see or read the decimal in front of the one. Likewise, the same applies for the digoxin dose. The leading zero in these cases verifies that the dose is a very small number—less than one.

Addition and Subtraction

Addition and subtraction of decimals has one basic rule: *Always line up the decimal points when adding or subtracting.*

■ **EXAMPLE 11**

22.6	124.342	156.43
14.407	34.2	− 35.2
+ 54.33	+ 4.17	121.23
91.337	162.712	

Multiplication

Multiplying decimals is the same as multiplying any other whole number. Once the answer is determined, you insert the decimal according to the total number of positions taken by all the decimals in the original numbers, counting from right to left.

■ **EXAMPLE 12**

4.236
× 2.41
10.20876

There are five decimal places total (three in the first number and, two in the second). Counting from the right, you would place the decimal point after the first zero and before the 2.

Division

In order to divide decimals, you must make them whole numbers before dividing them. To do this, you move the decimal point to the right until a whole number is made. If both numbers do not have the same amount of decimal places, you will move the decimal in the number with the largest amount of decimal places first. Next, count the number of places it was moved and then move the decimal in the second number the same number of positions, filling in the "extra" spots with zeros. Now you can perform the division.

■ EXAMPLE 13

$$\frac{4.234}{1.67} = 4234 \div 1670 = 2.5353$$

The decimal places in the numerator are three, so move it to the right that many places. The denominator has only two, so you will move it two places plus one more by putting a zero in that position.

Rounding

When you are multiplying and dividing decimals, your answer may have more decimal digits than your original numbers. For measurement of liquids, you will generally round to the nearest tenth. Tuberculin and insulin syringes allow you to measure to the nearest hundredth. Solid measurements can be accurately measured to the hundredth.

To perform this calculation, you will look at the number to the immediate right of the one you wish to round. If that number is four or less, it will remain the same. If the number to the right of the one you wish to round is five or higher, you will add one to that number.

■ EXAMPLE 14

Round to the nearest tenth.

14.234 → 14.2   The number to the immediate right of the "tenth" position is a 3, so the number in the "tenth" position remains the same (2).

1.5932 → 1.6   The number to the immediate right of the "tenth" position is a 9, so the number in the "tenth" position will increase by one.

When performing multiplication and division of decimals where the result is not being used for measuring purposes, then the rounding of the decimal will be determined by the equation itself. If you are multiplying a number with four decimal positions and another one with only two decimal positions, then the final answer will retain only two decimal positions. An equation's answer is only as accurate as the number with the least decimal positions.

■ **EXAMPLE 15**

Multiply the following.

3.5433 × 2.42 = 8.574786 = 8.57

The answer results in a number with six decimal positions. The first number has four decimal positions, and the second number has only two. Therefore, the answer can have only two decimal positions. Following the rules of rounding numbers from above, the four (4) is used to determine the rounding of the second decimal position (7). Since the number is less than five, it will remain the same.

Practice Problems 2.3

Round to the correct decimal position.

1. 23.4 × 42.87 =
2. 8.56 × 39.2 =
3. 146 × 15.58 =
4. 1.4756 × 2.4 =
5. 3.4 × 4.21 × 1.8 =
6. 4.56 ÷ 2.3 =
7. 45.98 ÷ 9.135 =
8. 7.34 ÷ 4.9 =
9. 5.3214 ÷ 3.87 =
10. 24 ÷ 4.34 =

Significant Figures

A significant figure is a digit of known value in a number that can be accurately measured. A number usually consists of one or several significant figures, or digits, plus one more digit that cannot be considered accurate but is needed to hold a position in the number. Consider the following rules when determining significant figures:

1. All leading zeros are not significant.
2. All zeros within (surrounded) by digits are significant.
3. Count all digits from left to right excluding leading zeros.
4. Zeros at the end of a digit may or may not be significant depending on the accuracy of the measuring tool.

■ **EXAMPLE 16**

Remember:
Leading zeros
NEVER count!

0.0125 = 3 significant figures (two leading zeros)

1.032 = 4 significant figures (zero within digits)

18,543 = 5 significant figures

4.34 = 3 significant figures

0.9 = 1 significant figure (leading zero)

Remember:
Trailing zeros may or may not count—it depends on the accuracy of the measurement.

3.0 = 1 significant figure

or

2 significant figures—*if* it is stated that the calculation is accurate to the "tenth" position

8.430 = 3 significant figures

Practice Problems 2.4

Determine the significant figures—final zeros are *not* significant.

1. 0.254
2. 1.085
3. 43.2
4. 2.0001
5. 3.0
6. 902
7. 5439.1
8. 1.2040
9. 22,432.2
10. 0.0003
11. 700
12. 0.019040

Round to three significant figures.

13. 57.82
14. 49.074
15. 0.5486
16. 0.00486
17. 1.438
18. 1.899

CHAPTER 2 QUIZ

Perform the following calculations. Simplify when possible.

1. $\dfrac{2}{4} + \dfrac{2}{3} =$

2. $\dfrac{4}{5} + \dfrac{7}{8} =$

3. $\dfrac{6}{20} + \dfrac{4}{10} + \dfrac{4}{5} =$

4. $\dfrac{9}{14} - \dfrac{3}{14} =$

5. $2\dfrac{5}{6} + 3\dfrac{1}{4} =$

6. $\dfrac{5}{6} \times \dfrac{3}{8} =$

7. $\dfrac{10}{75} \times \dfrac{20}{100} =$

8. $\dfrac{7}{15} \times \dfrac{3}{4} =$

9. $8 \div \dfrac{2}{3} =$

10. $3\dfrac{1}{3} \times 4\dfrac{1}{4} =$

11. $\dfrac{5}{9} + \dfrac{2}{9} =$

12. $\dfrac{2}{15} + \dfrac{8}{15} =$

13. $\dfrac{7}{8} - \dfrac{3}{4} =$

14. $\dfrac{5}{8} - \dfrac{1}{3} =$

15. $4\dfrac{2}{13} + 3\dfrac{7}{26} =$

16. $\dfrac{11}{14} \times \dfrac{1}{4} =$

17. $\dfrac{2}{3} \times \dfrac{1}{4} \times \dfrac{7}{8} =$

18. $\dfrac{5}{8} \div \dfrac{1}{2} =$

19. $\dfrac{2}{7} \div 4 =$

20. $6\dfrac{1}{4} \div 3\dfrac{1}{3} =$

Perform the following calculations. Round to the proper decimal position.

1. 23.6 + 42.87 =
2. 346.42 + 2.68 + 49.572 =
3. 423.73 − 284.6 =
4. 26.84 − 14.82 =
5. 3.1 × 6.82 =
6. 7.42 ÷ 3.6 =
7. 9.8624 ÷ 4.36 =
8. 17 ÷ 2.46 =
9. 5.62 × 3.9 =
10. 8.92 × 2.6 =

Determine the significant figures—final zeros are *not* significant.

1. 0.426
2. 3.028
3. 7326.4
4. 1.8604
5. 7.0

Round to three significant figures.

1. 52.083
2. 1.377
3. 0.6491
4. 1.888
5. 234.2

Ratio, Proportions, and Percents

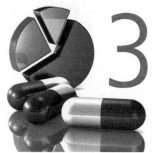

OBJECTIVES

- Define ratios, proportions, and percents
- Be able to interpret ratios, proportions, and percents
- Be able to convert ratios to percents
- Be able to convert percents to ratios
- Be able to convert percents to decimals
- Be able to perform calculations using ratios, proportion, and percents

RATIOS

Ratios represent the relationship between two numbers. Another way to define a ratio is the comparison of the magnitude of two like values (3:5; 2:7). They are written with a colon in between the two values. The ratio of 3:5 is read as follows: *three parts to five parts*. This ratio means that for every three parts of one value, five parts of the other value will be needed. Ratios are also written as fractions. In pharmacy, the fraction is the most common form of ratios. It is also the easiest format to perform calculations (see **Table 3.1**).

In pharmacy, you will see ratios representing the strengths of medications. The strength is a measure of the concentration of the drug per solid unit or the concentration of the drug in a solution. Solids are represented by tablets, ointments, creams, and powders. Tablets or capsules have a value of x per one (500 mg per tablet/capsule or 500:1). Ointments, creams, and powders are expressed in units per weight. The gram is the most common weight measure for solids (200 mg per 15 gm or 200:15). Liquids can be in oral or injectable form. Liquids are expressed as units of drug (weight or volume) per volume of liquid (mL). Oral liquids are usually expressed in concentrations per teaspoon (125 mg/5 mL). Injectable liquids are listed in a variety of ways, but often there will be a reference to a "per unit" ratio also (250 mg/10 mL or 25 mg/mL). This information is valuable. It helps to determine the amount of the medication needed for the desired dose. Most tablets and capsules are dispensed in whole units, but occasionally you might need to dispense partial ($\frac{1}{2}$ or $\frac{1}{4}$) tablets.

TABLE 3.1   **Ratio, Definition, and Fraction**

Ratio	Definition	Fraction
1:6	One part to six parts	$\frac{1}{6}$
2:9	Two parts to nine parts	$\frac{2}{9}$
3:20	Three parts to twenty parts	$\frac{3}{20}$
7:8	Seven parts to eight parts	$\frac{7}{8}$

■ **EXAMPLE 1**

Dispense Demeclomycin 250 mg tablet per dose. Pharmacy stocks 500 mg tablets.

The ratio for the tablet you have on hand is 500:1 or $\dfrac{500 \text{ mg}}{1 \text{ tab}}$

The ratio for the tablet you need is 250:x or $\dfrac{250 \text{ mg}}{x}$

The ratio to solve the problem would look like this: $\dfrac{500 \text{ mg}}{1 \text{ tab}} : \dfrac{250 \text{ mg}}{x}$

Liquid medications come in unit-dose form (each dose is individually packaged) or in bulk packages. Both types of packaging have the concentration (ratio) of the drug printed on it. When a liquid medication is ordered and the desired dose is available in a unit-dose package with the correct concentration, nothing else needs to be done from a calculation standpoint. When a medication is ordered and the drug is only available in bulk packaging, the desired dose must be calculated using the ratio (concentration) provided on the label. The same ratio formula used in Example 1 is used to solve this equation.

■ **EXAMPLE 2**

Dispense Oxybutnin 20 mg per dose. Pharmacy stocks 5 mg/5 mL, 1 pint bottles.

The ratio of the drug on hand is 5:5 or $\dfrac{5 \text{ mg}}{5 \text{ mL}}$

The ratio of the drug you need is 20:x or $\dfrac{20 \text{ mg}}{x}$

The ratio to solve the problem would look like this: $\dfrac{5 \text{ mg}}{5 \text{ mL}} = \dfrac{20 \text{ mg}}{x}$

Medication concentrations expressed in ratio form (a:b) can be read in three different ways depending on the form of the drug and the diluent (substance the drug is carried in or dissolved in). A drug that has a concentration of 1:1000 can mean one of the following:

1 g of drug per 1000 g of solid (cream/ointment/powder) = weight/weight (w/w)

1 g of drug per 1000 mL of liquid = weight/volume (w/v)

1 mL of drug per 1000 mL of liquid = volume/volume (v/v)

This concept is discussed further in Chapter 5.

Practice Problems 3.1

Convert the following ratios to fractions and simplify to the lowest term possible.

1. 3:9
2. 2:5
3. 5:20
4. 1:10
5. 6:7
6. 14:23
7. 3:4
8. 8:3
9. 1:18
10. 4:25

Convert the following fractions to ratios and simplify to the lowest term possible.

11. $\dfrac{3}{4}$
12. $\dfrac{4}{6}$
13. $\dfrac{1}{8}$
14. $\dfrac{2}{1000}$
15. $\dfrac{15}{30}$
16. $\dfrac{1}{10,000}$
17. $\dfrac{3}{9}$
18. $\dfrac{10}{12}$
19. $\dfrac{5}{9}$
20. $\dfrac{7}{49}$

Determine the ratio for the following drugs and simplify to the lowest term possible.

21. 750 mg tablet of clarithromycin
22. 10 mg capsule dicyclomine
23. 125 mg of amoxicillin in 5 mL
24. 300 mg of ranitidine in 2 mL
25. 20 mg of diphenhydramine in 1 g

Write a ratio equation for the following problems.

26. Dispense cimetidine 400 mg per dose; on hand is 200 mg tablets
27. Dispense 10 mg metoclopramide per dose; on hand is 5 mg/mL
28. Dispense 250 mg dicloxacillin per dose; on hand is 500 mg/5 mL

Define the following ratios.

29. 1:2000 w/w
30. 2:500 w/v

Remember:
A ratio can be expressed as a whole number (1:3) or as a fraction $\left(\frac{1}{3}\right)$.

PROPORTIONS

A proportion is defined as an expression of two equal ratios. A ratio can be expressed in whole numbers separated by a colon or as a fraction. A proportion, therefore, can be expressed as two ratios (numerals or fractions) separated by two colons. It can also be expressed with an equal sign instead of the two colons.

■ **EXAMPLE 3**

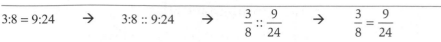

$$3:8 = 9:24 \quad \rightarrow \quad 3:8 :: 9:24 \quad \rightarrow \quad \frac{3}{8} :: \frac{9}{24} \quad \rightarrow \quad \frac{3}{8} = \frac{9}{24}$$

Since proportions are a symbol of equality between two ratios, you need to verify that they are, in fact, equal. Proportions have a simple rule to verify that equality. In order to do this, the components of a proportion should be defined.

A proportion, whether it is in numeral form or in fraction form, has two sets of values: the means and the extremes. In numeral form, the outside values are the extremes and the middle values are the means. One way to remember which set of number represents the means and which set represents the extremes is to relate the word *extreme* with *extremities*. Extremities are on the outside or far ends (e.g., arms/legs).

■ **EXAMPLE 4**

Means and Extremes.

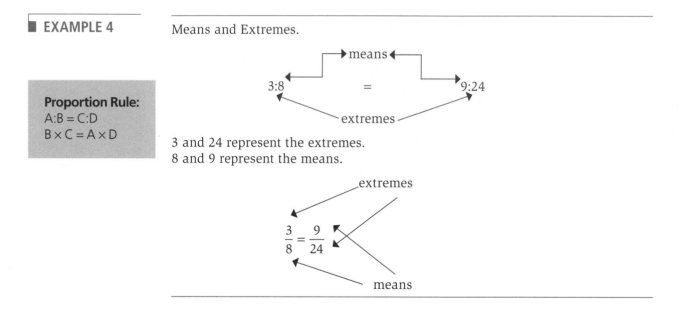

Proportion Rule:
A:B = C:D
B × C = A × D

3 and 24 represent the extremes.
8 and 9 represent the means.

Fraction ratios:

> **means** = denominator of the first ratio and the numerator of the second ratio

> **extremes** = numerator of the first ratio and the denominator of the second ratio

If a proportion is equal, the product of the means will always equal the product of the extremes. You can verify this by multiplying the means together and then multiplying the extremes together.

8 × 9 (means) = 3 × 24 (extremes)
            72 = 72

By understanding ratios and proportions, almost any problem can be solved when calculating pharmacy dosages. This method of problem solving is called the **ratio-proportion method**. As long as three of the four values in the proportion are known, the answer x can be determined. The ratio must be set up with the numerators sharing the same unit of measure and the denominators sharing the same unit of measure. By using simple algebra principles, the problem can be solved. Check the answer by applying the proportion rule: the product of the means equals the product of the extremes.

■ **EXAMPLE 5**

A patient needs 150 mg of medication. The pharmacy stocks 250 mg/5 mL strength.

Set up your ratio: $\dfrac{250 \text{ mg}}{5 \text{ mL}} = \dfrac{150 \text{ mg}}{x}$ You know three of the four values.

Cross multiply: $(250 \text{ mg})x = (150 \text{ mg} \times 5 \text{ mL})$ $A \times D = B \times C$

Divide: $\dfrac{150 \text{ mg} \times 5 \text{ mL}}{250 \text{ mg}}$ Solve for x.

Solution: $x = 3 \text{ mL}$

Check: $\dfrac{250 \text{ mg}}{5 \text{ mL}} = \dfrac{150 \text{ mg}}{3 \text{ mL}} = (250 \text{ mg} \times 3 \text{ mL}) = (150 \text{ mg} \times 5 \text{ mL})$

(extremes) 750 mg = 750 mg (means)

■ **EXAMPLE 6**

A patient needs 300 mg of medication. The pharmacy stocks 250 mg/5 mL strength.

1. $\dfrac{250 \text{ mg}}{5 \text{ mL}} = \dfrac{300 \text{ mg}}{x}$

2. $(250 \text{ mg})x = (300 \text{ mg} \times 5 \text{ mL})$

3. $\dfrac{300 \text{ mg} \times 5 \text{ mL}}{250 \text{ mg}} = x$

4. $x = 6 \text{ mL}$

5. $\dfrac{250 \text{ mg}}{5 \text{ mL}} = \dfrac{300 \text{ mg}}{6 \text{ mL}} = (250 \text{ mg} \times 6 \text{ mL}) = (300 \text{ mg} \times 5 \text{ mL})$

6. 1500 mg = 1500 mg

■ **EXAMPLE 7**

A patient weighs 66 pounds; convert this to kilograms.

1. $\dfrac{1 \text{ kg}}{2.2 \text{ lbs}} = \dfrac{x \text{ kg}}{66 \text{ lbs}}$

2. $(2.2 \text{ lbs})x = (1 \text{ kg} \times 66 \text{ lbs})$

3. $\dfrac{1 \text{ kg} \times 66 \text{ lbs}}{2.2 \text{ kg}} = x$

4. $x = 30 \text{ kg}$

Ratio-Proportion Rule:

Ratio-Proportion Rule:
1. Must know three of four values in a ratio.
2. Numerators must have same unit of measure.
3. Denominators must have same unit of measure.

Practice Problems 3.2

Solve for x.

1. $\dfrac{4}{12} = \dfrac{x}{3}$

2. $\dfrac{x}{42} = \dfrac{1}{7}$

3. $\dfrac{0.5}{4} = \dfrac{x}{16}$

4. $\dfrac{250}{5} = \dfrac{375}{x}$

5. $\dfrac{7}{10} = \dfrac{x}{9}$

6. $\dfrac{21}{x} = \dfrac{105}{5}$

7. $\dfrac{330}{5} = \dfrac{495}{x}$

8. $\dfrac{x}{50} = \dfrac{20}{250}$

9. $\dfrac{0.5}{1} = \dfrac{6}{x}$

10. $\dfrac{375}{12} = \dfrac{x}{16}$

Convert the following weights using the proportion rule.

11. 450 mg = x g

12. 0.95 g = x mg

13. 2450 mg = x g

14. 2.75 mg = x mcg

15. 540 mcg = x mg

16. 65 lbs = x kg

17. 240 kg = x lbs

18. 120 kg = x lbs

19. 132 lbs = x kg

20. 22 lbs = x kg

Use the proportion rule to solve for needed dosage in the following problems.

21. A prescription calls for 225 mg dose of amoxicillin every 6 hr for 10 days. The pharmacy carries 125 mg/5 mL concentration.

    a. How much is needed for each dose?

    b. How much is needed to fill the entire prescription?

22. Heparin comes in 5000 units/mL concentration; the patient needs a dose of 2000 units. How many mLs are needed?

23. A patient needs 550 mg of amikacin. The pharmacy carries 500 mg/2 mL vials. How much is needed for this dose?

24. An IV solution needs 35 mEq of potassium added. The pharmacy carries 50 mL vials with a concentration of 2 mEq/mL. How much is needed for this dose?

25. A prescription calls for 500 mg of erythromycin. The pharmacy only carries 250 mg tablets. How many will be dispensed for each dose?

26. A physician orders furosemide 50 mg IV now for a patient. The pharmacy carries 20 mg/2 mL concentration. How much will you dispense for this dose?

27. You receive a prescription for albuterol 4 mg twice a day for 14 days. The pharmacy carries 2 mg/5 mL concentration in pint bottles.

    a. How much will the patient take per dose?

    b. How much will you dispense to fill the entire prescription?

28. Propranolol 40 mg tablets are ordered for a patient. The pharmacy is out of 40 mg tablets and has only 80 mg tablets available. How many tablets will be dispensed for a 40 mg dose?

29. An infant needs 10 mg/kg of an antibiotic. The infant weighs 11 lbs. The antibiotic is available in 100 mg/10 mL concentration.

    a. How much does the infant weigh in kg?

    b. What is the dose needed for the infant?

    c. How many mLs of the antibiotic are needed for this dose?

30. A patient has a prescription for clindamycin 300 mg four times a day for 14 days. The pharmacy only carries the 150 mg capsules.

    a. How many capsules are needed per dose?

    b. How many capsules are needed daily?

    c. How many capsules are needed for the entire prescription?

PERCENTS

The word percent means "per 100." When a number is represented as a percent (%), it is a relationship between that number and 100. In other words, a percent is a part, or fraction, of a whole. Percents are represented in many different forms. They can be fractions, ratios, or decimals (see **Table 3.2**).

An 82% represents 82 parts of a total of 100 parts. Its decimal equivalent is 0.82 and its fraction is $\frac{82}{100}$. The decimal is made by simply moving the decimal point two positions to the left.

■ **EXAMPLE 8**

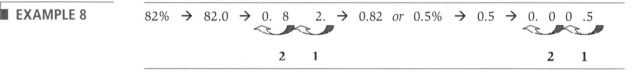

82% → 82.0 → 0. 8   2. → 0.82 *or* 0.5% → 0.5 → 0. 0 0 .5

                    2   1   2   1

The fraction is made by placing the percent over 100.

■ **EXAMPLE 9**

82% = $\frac{82}{100}$ 0.5% = $\frac{0.5}{100}$

The ratio is made by placing a colon between the number and 100.

TABLE 3.2   **Different Forms of Percents**

Percent	Decimal	Fraction	Ratio
32%	0.32	32/100	32:100
5%	0.05	5/100	5:100
0.75%	0.0075	0.75/100	0.75:100
110%	1.10	110/100	110:100

■ EXAMPLE 10

$$82\% = 82{:}100 \qquad\qquad 0.5\% = 0.5{:}100$$

The percent is used most often to express the concentration of intravenous (IV) solutions and topical medications (creams and ointments). This can also be called a percent strength. Again, it describes the amount of drug contained in a specific volume (liquid or solid). An IV solution containing 5% dextrose has 5 g of dextrose for every 100 mL of solution. It could also be translated as 5 g/100 mL, 0.05 or 5:100. An ointment that contains 0.1% triamcinolone has 0.1 g of triamcinolone for every 100 g of ointment. This translates to 0.1 g/100 mL, 0.001, or 0.1:100 as a fraction, decimal, or ratio, respectively. The larger the percent number, the stronger the solution will be. A 10% solution (10 g/100 mL) is much stronger than a 1% solution (1 g/100 mL).

CONVERSIONS

The percent is the most common way to represent drug strength or concentration. This means you sometimes need to convert a ratio, fraction, or decimal to a percent.

Ratio to Percent

The format of a ratio is the drug (solute) in relation to the solvent (liquid or solution). Therefore, the position of the numbers is important. A ratio of 5:1 is not the same as a ratio of 1:5. A ratio of 5:1 means that there are five parts of drug to one part of solute. This is much different than 1:5, which represents one part of drug to five parts of solute. To convert these ratios to a percent, divide the first number by the second number and then multiply that answer by 100.

■ EXAMPLE 11

$$4{:}1 = \frac{4}{1} \times 100\% = 4 \times 100\% = 400\%$$

$$1{:}4 = \frac{1}{4} \times 100\% = \frac{100\%}{4} = 25\%$$

$$0.5{:}4 = \frac{0.5}{4} \times 100\% = \frac{0.5 \times 100\%}{4} = 12.5\%$$

Decimal to Percent

The process to convert a decimal to a percent can be done two different ways. Likewise, the process can be reversed to go from percent to decimal format. The first way is to move the decimal point two positions to the right. The second is to multiply the decimal by 100.

■ **EXAMPLE 12**

0.62 → 0. 6 2. → 62%   1.42 → 1. 4 2. → 142%

   1   **2**   **1**   **2**

0.62 × 100% = 62%   1.42 × 100% = 142%

0.032 × 100 = 3.2%

Percent to decimal would be moving the decimal two positions to the left as shown in Example 8, or dividing the percent number by 100 (22% → 22 ÷ 100 = 0.22).

Practice Problems 3.3

Convert the following ratios to percents.

1. 2:300
2. 3:4
3. 1:1000
4. 1:5
5. 6:10

Convert the following percents to ratios and simplify to the lowest form.

6. 3%
7. 42%
8. 0.5%
9. 1.6%
10. 150%

Convert the following fractions to percents.

11. $\frac{5}{7}$
12. $\frac{2}{8}$
13. $\frac{14}{52}$
14. $\frac{0.4}{2}$
15. $\frac{3}{4}$

Convert the following percents to fractions and simplify to the lowest form.

16. 24%
17. 0.25%
18. 140%
19. 1.65%
20. 2%

Calculate the following percents.

21. 5% of 50
22. 20% of 60
23. 18% of 42
24. 110% of 75
25. 0.5% of 80

CHAPTER 3 QUIZ

Convert the following ratios to fractions and simplify when possible.

1. 4:10
2. 3:15
3. 6:50
4. 40:1000
5. 2:7

Convert the following fractions to ratios and simplify when possible.

1. $\dfrac{120}{700}$
2. $\dfrac{1}{9}$
3. $\dfrac{5}{40}$
4. $\dfrac{1}{1000}$
5. $\dfrac{6}{240}$

Convert the following percents to ratios and simplify when possible.

1. 20%
2. 4%
3. 58%
4. 0.4%
5. 1.5%

Convert the following ratios to percents.

1. 2:3
2. 1:500
3. 4:10
4. 15:40
5. 1:1000

Convert the following fractions to percents.

1. $\dfrac{5}{7}$

2. $\dfrac{42}{100}$

3. $\dfrac{3}{10}$

4. $\dfrac{9}{20}$

5. $\dfrac{0.8}{10}$

Convert the following percents to fractions and simplify when possible.

1. 52%

2. 3%

3. 110%

4. 0.4%

5. 3.7%

Solve the following proportions.

1. $\dfrac{9}{42} = \dfrac{x}{126}$ 6. $\dfrac{125}{5} = \dfrac{400}{x}$

2. $\dfrac{14}{x} = \dfrac{70}{85}$ 7. $\dfrac{1500}{50} = \dfrac{x}{10}$

3. $\dfrac{3}{5} = \dfrac{24}{x}$ 8. $\dfrac{400}{5} = \dfrac{x}{20}$

4. $\dfrac{82}{x} = \dfrac{41}{68}$ 9. $\dfrac{40}{2} = \dfrac{180}{x}$

5. $\dfrac{x}{110} = \dfrac{80}{440}$ 10. $\dfrac{1000}{10} = \dfrac{300}{x}$

Solve the following problems.

1. Diazepam comes in 5 mg/mL concentration. The dose is 3 mg. How many mLs are needed for the dose?

2. The patient needs 450 mg of clindamycin. The pharmacy stocks 300 mg/2 mL concentration. How many mLs are needed for the dose?

3. An antibiotic suspension is available in 500 mg/5 mL concentration. The dose is 150 mg four times a day.

    a. How many mLs are needed for one dose?

    b. How many mLs are need for one day?

4. How many 300 mg doses can be made from 5400 mg?

5. Amoxicillin is available in 250 mg/5 mL concentration. A patient needs 375 mg four times a day for 14 days.

    a. How many mLs will be needed for one dose?

    b. How many mLs will be needed for the entire 14 days?

6. The pharmacy has an order for gentamicin 170 mg. The concentration of the stock solution is 40 mg/mL. How much is needed for this dose?

7. Dexamethasone elixir is available in 4 mg/5 mL concentration. The patient needs a 10 mg dose daily for 7 days.

    a. How many mLs is a 10 mg dose?

    b. How much is needed for the full 7 days?

8. Codeine 40 mg is ordered. The stock vial is 60 mg/2 mL. How many mLs are needed for the dose?

9. Ferrous sulfate comes in 220 mg/5 mL concentration. How many mg are in 7.5 mL?

10. Potassium chloride liquid is available in 20 mEq/15 mL concentration. The patient needs 50 mEq two times a day.

    a. How much will be used for one dose?

    b. How much will be used daily?

Liquid Measures

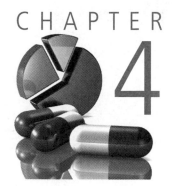

OBJECTIVES

- Define density
- Define specific gravity
- Be able to calculate density
- Be able to calculate specific gravity

INTRODUCTION

Density and specific gravity are not often used for calculation purposes in pharmacy. However, knowing what these are and how they can be used is helpful information. When density or specific gravity are used, they are most often associated with compounding and in complicated IV admixtures. The information is listed on medication labels, and some manufacturers are required to list that information on their packaging.

DENSITY

Density is described as the mass per unit of volume of a particular substance. It is normally written as **grams/cc (mL)**. The standard, or constant, that it is measured against is the mass of 1 mL of water at 4°C. This means that the density of water is 1 g/mL. The density for substances, usually chemicals, is found on the label. IV solutions also have the density listed. This may be used to calibrate IV admixture machines. Some of these machines determine the necessary volume of an IV solution based on its density. Some use the specific gravity.

The formula for calculating density is mass divided by volume.

$$\text{density} = \frac{\text{mass}}{\text{volume}}$$

▪ **EXAMPLE 1**

Liquid A has a volume of 20 mL and weighs 24 g. Find the density.

$$D = \frac{24\ g}{20\ mL} = 1.2\ g/mL$$

Liquid B weighs 50 g and the container holds 120 mL. Find the density.

$$D = \frac{50\ g}{120\ mL} = 0.42\ g/mL$$

SPECIFIC GRAVITY

Specific gravity is the ratio of the weight of a liquid or solid in relation to the weight of an equal volume or mass of water. It is expressed as a decimal. If this ratio is less than one (0.82), then the substance is lighter than water. If this ratio is more than one (1.4), then the substance is heavier than water. This is best seen in tubes of colored liquid that have been layered. Each color liquid has a different specific gravity. The liquid with the smallest specific gravity number is on top, and the liquid with the highest specific gravity number is on the bottom. Gases also have specific gravity, and their ratio is determined by using hydrogen as the standard instead of water.

In pharmacies with a high volume of total parenteral nutrition (TPN) solutions, specific gravity is used to measure the multiple ingredients' volumes. TPNs have multiple additives, and two to three main solutions are combined to provide intravenous nutrition to patients. These pharmacies have an IV admixture compounding machine that operates by combining set volumes of fluid based on the known specific gravity of the solutions and additives needed.

The formula for specific gravity is the weight of the substance divided by the weight of an equal volume of water.

$$\text{Specific gravity} = \frac{\text{weight (liquid/solid)}}{\text{weight = volume (H}_2\text{O)}}$$

We know that water has a mass (weight) of 1 g/mL based on the definition of the gram. One g is the mass of 1 mL of water at 4°C.

▪ **EXAMPLE 2**

Determine the specific gravity of 20 mL of an acid with a mass of 42 g.

$$\text{Specific gravity} = \frac{42\ g}{20\ g\ (20\ mL - H_2O\ weight)} = 2.1$$

The specific gravity of this acid is 2.1.

Specific gravity is a constant. It will always be the same for any given substance. This means that if the specific gravity for an acid A is 2.4, then it will always be 2.4. It does not change with volume or mass. Ten mL has the same specific gravity as 50 mL. **Table 4.1** has some common liquids listed with their specific gravities.

When the substances listed with a specific gravity above water are added to water, they will rise to the top and float on top of the water with a clear line of separation. The substances with a specific gravity listed below water will settle below the water, allowing the water to float on top of the substance.

TABLE 4.1   **Specific Gravities**

Substance	Specific Gravity
Isopropyl Alcohol	0.78
Alcohol	0.81
Olive Oil	0.91
Castor Oil	0.96
Water (Constant)	**1.00**
Liquid Phenol	1.07
Glycerin	1.25
Hydrochloric Acid	1.37
Mercury	13.60

CHAPTER 4 QUIZ

Round answers to the second decimal place.

1. What is the specific gravity of a liquid with a volume of 15 mL and a mass of 30 g?
2. What is the specific gravity of an acid with a mass of 62 g and a volume of 40 mL?
3. What is the specific gravity of a solution with a volume of 120 mL and a mass of 60 g?
4. What is the specific gravity of 2 oz of glycerin with a mass of 78 g? (*Hint:* 1 oz = 30 mL)
5. What is the specific gravity of 1 L of phenol with a mass of 1450 g? (*Hint:* 1 L = 1000 mL)
6. Alcohol has a specific gravity of 0.81. What is the volume if the mass is 125 g?
7. What is the mass of mercury if the specific gravity is 13.6 and the volume is 50 mL?
8. A bottle of cough syrup weighs 16 oz and has a volume of 240 mL. What is the specific gravity? (*Hint:* 1 oz = 30 g)
9. The mass of antacid liquid is 360 g with a specific gravity of 1.6. What is the volume?
10. The volume of a cleaning agent that has a specific gravity of 1.2 is 946 mL. What is the mass?

Concentrations

CHAPTER 5

OBJECTIVES

- Be able to determine weight/weight concentrations
- Be able to determine volume/volume concentrations
- Be able to determine weight/volume concentrations
- Be able to perform calculations using ratio strength
- Be able to perform calculations using percent strength

WEIGHT/WEIGHT

The concentration of a medication that is listed as % w/w is a proportion of the active ingredient (solute) in relation to the inactive ingredient, or carrier (solvent). It is most often used to describe solid or semisolid products because they are measured based on their mass or weight. Ointments, creams, gels, lotions, and some tablets or capsules will have their dosage strength listed in % w/w form.

The expression of % w/w on a drug label means x g/100 g of solute to solvent, or medication in a carrier. When you see percent (%) used to describe the strength of a solid or semisolid product, it carries the same meaning as % w/w. The most common place to see the designation % w/w is on bulk chemicals.

Bacitracin ointment 0.5% has 0.5 g of active ingredient, bacitracin, in every 100 g of ointment. This is important to understand. This information can help determine the total amount of active drug in any given quantity dispensed.

■ EXAMPLE 1

Remember:
%strength =
x g/100 g of drug.

Betamethasone 0.1% cream, 120 g tube is dispensed to a patient. How much betamethasone is in the 120 g tube?

$$\frac{0.1\,\text{g}}{100\,\text{g}} = \frac{x}{120\,\text{g}}$$

$x = (0.1 \times 120) \div 100 = 0.12\,\text{g}$

▪ **EXAMPLE 2**

A patient is prescribed diphenhydramine 2% cream. The directions ask for 50 mg per dose. How much is needed per dose?

$$\frac{2\ g}{100\ g} = \frac{50\ mg}{x} \left(\frac{2\ g = 2000\ mg}{100\ g} = \frac{50\ mg}{x} \right)$$

$$x = (50\ mg \times 100\ mg) \div 2000\ mg = 2.5\ g$$

▪ **EXAMPLE 3**

A prescription asks for 60 g of lidocaine 4% w/w ointment. How much lidocaine 10% w/w powder is needed to compound this prescription?

$$\frac{4\ g}{100\ g} = \frac{x}{60\ g}$$

$$x = (4g \times 60\ g) \div 100\ g = 24\ g \quad \text{amount of lidocaine needed in the entire 60 g}$$

$$\frac{10\ g}{100\ g} = \frac{2.4\ g}{x}$$

$$x = (2.4\ g \times 100\ g) \div 10\ g = 24\ g \quad \text{10% lidocaine to be added to the ointment base}$$

To obtain a total weight of 60 g, subtract the 24 g of lidocaine from 60 g to obtain the amount of ointment base needed to complete the prescription.

Lidocaine 10% = 24 g
Ointment base = 36 g

VOLUME/VOLUME

Volume/volume concentration (% v/v) describes the concentration of a liquid dissolved in another liquid. An example might be diluting chlorine (bleach) in water—liquid in a liquid. Acetic acid is another liquid that is often diluted in either water or saline. Alcohol is yet another liquid dissolved into another liquid. A concentration of 12% v/v of phenol means that there is 12 mL of phenol in every 100 mL of solution. Again, as in the % w/w designation, this is often seen only on chemical reagents. These are concentrated solutions used for the sole purpose of dilution or addition to other products. Many of the agents are very caustic in full strength and are never used without further dilution.

▪ **EXAMPLE 4**

An alcohol solution is labeled as 10% v/v. How much alcohol is in 200 mL?

$$\frac{10\ mL}{100\ mL} = \frac{x}{200\ mL}$$

$$x = (10\ mL \times 200\ mL) \div 100\ mL = 20\ mL$$

■ **EXAMPLE 5**   20 mL of acetic acid is diluted with 80 mL of sterile water. What is the % v/v?

$$\frac{20 \text{ mL}}{100 \text{ mL}} = x\%$$

$x = 20 \text{ mL}/100 \text{ mL} = 0.2 \times 100 = 20\% \text{ v/v}$

The 20 mL represents the medication in the solution.

The 100 mL represents the total amount of liquid (20 + 80).

Multiply the answer by 100 to obtain a percent quantity.

(24 mL in 120 mL will produce the same concentration—24 mL/120 mL = 20%).

■ **EXAMPLE 6**   Dilute 150 mL of chlorine in 600 mL of sterile water. What is the % v/v?

$$\frac{150 \text{ mL}}{750 \text{ mL}} = x\%$$

$x = 150 \text{ mL}/750 \text{ mL} = 0.2 \times 100 = 20\% \text{ v/v}$

WEIGHT/VOLUME

Weight/volume concentration describes the concentration of a solid dissolved in a liquid. IV solutions are an example of weight/volume concentration. They are expressed as % w/v, or x g/100 mL. An IV solution of D5%W (5% w/v) has 5 g/100 mL of dextrose.

■ **EXAMPLE 7**   How many milliliters of a 5% solution can be made from 250 g of dextrose?

$$\frac{5 \text{ g}}{100 \text{ mL}} = \frac{250 \text{ g}}{x}$$

$x = (250 \text{ g} \times 100 \text{ mL}) \div 5 \text{ g} = 5000 \text{ mL}$

■ **EXAMPLE 8**   A prescription calls for 120 mL of a 2% gentamicin solution. How much gentamicin powder is needed?

$$\frac{2 \text{ g}}{100 \text{ mL}} = \frac{x}{120 \text{ mL}}$$

$x = (2 \text{ g} \times 120 \text{ mL}) \div 100 \text{ mL} = 2.4 \text{ g}$

Practice Problems 5.1

1. How much tobramycin powder should be added to 240 g of an ointment base to obtain 4% w/w?

2. What is the % v/v concentration of 50 mL phenol added to 750 mL sterile water? (*Hint:* Remember that the fraction is volume of drug over total [final] volume.)

3. How many grams of clindamycin 3% ointment can be made from 500 g of clindamycin powder?

4. What is the % w/v of a solution with a concentration of 50 mg/mL?

5. A stock acid has a concentration of 50% v/v. How many milliliters will be needed to make 240 mL of a 2% solution?

6. An IV containing dextrose has a concentration of 70% w/v. How many grams of dextrose are in 600 mL?

7. What is the percent strength of a promethazine syrup made from 50 g of promethazine powder in 480 mL?

8. What is the % w/v of a ferrous sulfate solution of 300 mg/5 mL?

9. How many grams of dextrose are needed to make 3000 mL of a 5% w/v solution?

10. How many grams of talc should be used to prepare 500 g of an 8% w/w gel?

RATIO STRENGTH

Ratio strength represents the concentration of weak solutions. It is expressed in ratio form (*x:y*). A percent strength can be converted to a ratio strength and vice versa. Calculations can be performed in ratio format or converted to percent strength.

A solution with a concentration of 5% translates to 5:100 in ratio strength notation. When writing ratio strengths, the first number should be 1, so you need to reduce the ratio to its smallest denomination. A ratio of 5:100 reduces to a ratio of 1:20. These ratios read as follows: five parts to 100 parts or one part to 20 parts.

The rules are similar to those of % w/w, % w/v, and % v/v. If the product is a solid, then a ratio of 1:1000 would mean there is 1 g of solute to 1000 g of solvent/carrier. If the product is a liquid, it represents either a solid in liquid or a liquid in liquid. These translate to 1 g of solid to 1000 mL of liquid or 1 mL of liquid in 1000 mL of liquid, respectively.

■ **EXAMPLE 9**

Convert 0.05% to ratio strength.

$$\frac{0.05}{100} = \frac{1}{x}$$

$x = (1 \times 100)/0.05 = 2000 = 1{:}2000$

■ **EXAMPLE 10**

Convert 0.8% to ratio strength.

$$\frac{0.8}{100} = \frac{1}{x}$$
$$x = (1 \times 100)/0.8 = 125 = 1{:}125$$

■ **EXAMPLE 11**

Convert 1:2000 to percent strength.

$$\frac{1}{2000} = \frac{x\%}{100\%}$$
$$x = (1 \times 100)/2000 = 0.05\%$$

This information is also useful when percent strength or ratio strength needs to be converted to mg/mL (see **Table 5.1**). Many cardiac medication dosages are listed as ratio strengths (epinephrine 1:1000) or percent strengths (lidocaine 2%). Often orders are written for mg/mL dosages so conversion must be done. Remember that percent strength is x g/100 mL, so further conversion to milligrams is necessary.

■ **EXAMPLE 12**

Remember: Convert grams to milligrams for final calculations.

A patient needs 50 mg of lidocaine. The stock solution is 2% w/v.

$$\frac{2 \text{ g}}{100 \text{ mL}} = \frac{2000 \text{ mg}}{100 \text{ mL}} = \frac{50 \text{ mg}}{x}$$
$$x = (50 \text{ mg} \times 100 \text{ mL})/2000 \text{ mg} = 2.5 \text{ mL}$$

TABLE 5.1   Common Ratio to Percent Conversions

Ratio Strength	Fraction	Percent Strength
1:100	1/1 % (1/100)	1%
1:200	1/2 % (1/200)	0.5%
1:500	1/5 % (1/500)	0.2%
4:500	4/5 % (4/500)	0.8%
1:1000	1/10 % (1/1000)	0.1%
1:3500	1/35 % (1/3500)	0.028%
1:5000	1/50 % (1/5000)	0.02%
1:10,000	1/100 % (1/10,000)	0.01%

Assume the last two zeros are %, and place the remaining numbers in fraction form.

■ **EXAMPLE 13**

A patient needs 0.2 mg of adrenaline. The stock solution is 1:2000.

$$\frac{1 \text{ g}}{2000 \text{ mL}} = \frac{1000 \text{ mg}}{2000 \text{ mL}} = \frac{0.2 \text{ mg}}{x}$$

$x = (0.2 \text{ mg} \times 2000 \text{ mL})/1000 \text{ mg} = 0.4 \text{ mL}$

Practice Problems 5.2

1. Convert 0.25% to ratio strength.
2. Convert 1:200 to percent strength.
3. Convert 1:2500 to percent strength.
4. Convert 0.0125% to ratio strength.
5. Convert 1:10,000 to mg/mL.
6. Convert 4% to mg/mL.
7. A 30 mL vial of epinephrine 1:1000 contains how many milligrams of epinephrine?
8. What is the ratio strength of a 4 mg/mL solution?
9. Midazolam is available in 5 mg/mL strength. What is its ratio strength?
10. An anesthesiologist requests a solution with 3% cocaine and 1:4000 adrenaline for nasal application. How many milligrams of each solution will be needed for a 30 mL vial?

CHAPTER 5 QUIZ

Determine the total milligrams in each of the following medications.

1. Clindamycin 2% w/w cream 15 g tube
2. Gentamicin 0.1% w/w ointment 20 g tube
3. Metronidazole 0.5% w/w cream 45 g tube
4. Dextrose 50% w/v solution 750 mL
5. Iodine 14% w/v solution 120 mL
6. Zinc oxide 3% w/w ointment 454 g
7. Sodium chloride 23.4% w/v solution 60 mL

Determine the total milliliters of each medication in solution.

1. Alcohol 12% v/v 240 mL
2. Albuterol 0.04% v/v inhalation solution 300 mL
3. Thymol 0.05% solution in 250 mL

Calculate the percent strength.

1. Dextrose 70 g in 500 mL
2. Sodium chloride 12 g in 400 mL
3. Lidocaine ointment 30 g in 480 g
4. Nitroglycerin ointment 1.2 g in 60 g

5. Amikacin 500 mg/mL
6. Promethazine 50 mg/mL
7. 1:250
8. 1:400
9. 1:1000
10. Powder X 150 g dissolved in 1000 mL
11. Erythromycin 6 g in 120 g
12. Tobramycin 3 mg/mL

Calculate the ratio strength.

1. Betamethasone 0.01%
2. Midazolam 5 mg/mL
3. 2.5%
4. 0.8%
5. 1 mg/0.5 mL
6. Timolol 0.02%

Solve the following problems.

1. Dissolve 2400 mg of tobramycin powder in 120 mL. What is the %w/v?
2. Combine 50 g of zinc oxide with 400 g of an ointment base. What is the %w/w?
3. Add 150 mL water to 7.5 g of amoxicillin powder. What is the percent strength?
4. How many milliliters of phenol and diluent must be combined to create a solution of 12%v/v 1000 mL?
5. How much silver nitrate is needed to make 4 L of a 0.5% solution?

Dilutions

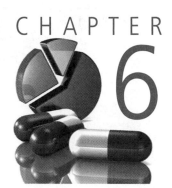

OBJECTIVES

- Be able to define a stock solution
- Be able to calculate dilution concentrations
- Be able to determine dilutions of liquids
- Be able to determine dilutions of solids
- Be able to perform allegation calculations

STOCK SOLUTIONS/SOLIDS

Stock solutions or solids are generally concentrated solutions or solids that are used to prepare weaker ones. Stock solutions or solid concentrations are often expressed as ratio strengths w/v or w/w (1:400 w/v) but can also be expressed as a percent strength w/v or w/w (50% w/v). Dilution of these concentrated solutions or solids creates a smaller concentration in a higher volume that will allow for easier, more accurate measurement of a desired dose.

A solution that has a concentration 50% (50 g/100 mL) and has the volume doubled now has a concentration of 25% (25 g/100 mL). The amount of medication (or solute) in the solution did not change, only the volume of the liquid (diluent). This means that the same amount of solute is now in twice as much diluent, creating a weaker solution. The same would be true for a solid product (ointment or creams). A cream with a percent strength of 18% (18 g/100 g) and a weight of 20 g that is combined with an additional 20 g of cream base would now have a percent strength of 9% (9 g/100 g).

When performing calculations to create a more dilute product, the shortest route is not always the best. It is more important to be accurate, so that may mean more steps in the calculation. Remembering two key rules can help simplify the process.

1. Ratio strengths should be converted to percent strengths for easier calculations. The ratio strength 1:500 = 0.2%.
2. Proportions (20:5) or fractions (6/30) should be simplified to their lowest form. The ratio 20:5 = 4:1 and the fraction $\frac{6}{30} = \frac{1}{5}$.

▪ **EXAMPLE 1**

How many milliliters of 1:500 w/v solution is needed to make 3 L of a 1:2000 w/v solution?

Convert ratios to percents: $1{:}500 = \dfrac{1}{500} = \dfrac{x}{100\%}$

$x = 0.2\% = 1{:}2000 = \dfrac{1}{2000} = \dfrac{x}{100\%}$

$x = 0.05\% \quad \dfrac{0.2\%}{0.05\%} = \dfrac{3000\text{ mL (3 L)}}{x}$

$x = (3000\text{ mL} \times 0.05\%) \div 0.2\% = 750\text{ mL}$

750 mL of the concentrated solution is added to 2250 mL of the diluent to obtain 3 L total volume with a concentration of 1:2000.

▪ **EXAMPLE 2**

How many grams of zinc oxide 10% ointment is needed to make 2400 g of a 3% concentration ointment?

$3\% = \dfrac{3\text{ g}}{100\text{ g}} = \dfrac{x}{2400\text{ g}}$

$x = (3\text{ g} \times 2400\text{ g}) \div 100\text{ g} = 72\text{ g}$, 72 g of zinc in 2400 g of a 3% concentration

$10\% = \dfrac{10\text{ g}}{100\text{ g}}$ so $\dfrac{10\text{ g}}{100\text{ g}} = \dfrac{72\text{ g}}{x}$

$x = (72\text{ g} \times 100\text{ g}) \div 10\text{ g} = 720\text{ g}$ of 10% zinc is needed

720 g of 10% zinc is added to 1680 g of ointment base for a total weight of 2400 g.

LIQUID DILUTIONS

Diluting liquids changes the concentration of that liquid. Since three of the four components are already known, the concentration of the new solution can be determined by using the proportion rule. This procedure can also be used to determine how much product (weaker strength) can be made from a known amount of a higher concentration.

▪ **EXAMPLE 3**

What is the new concentration (% strength) of a dextrose 70% 500 mL solution diluted to 2000 mL?

$70\% = \dfrac{70\text{ g}}{100\text{ mL}} = \dfrac{x}{500\text{ mL}}$

$x = (70\text{ g} \times 500\text{ mL}) \div 100\text{ mL} = 350\text{ g}$ total grams dextrose in 500 mL

$\dfrac{350\text{ g}}{2000\text{ mL}} = \dfrac{x}{100\text{ mL}}$

$x = (350\text{ g} \times 100\text{ mL}) \div 2000\text{ mL} = 17.5\text{ g} = 17.5\%$

This problem can also be solved by using the following formula:

Q1 (quantity 1) × C1 (concentration 1) = Q2 (quantity 2) × C2 (concentration 2)

The quantity 1 (Q1) and concentration 1 (C1) represents what is being diluted or changed. The quantity 2 (Q2) and concentration 2 (C2) represents the end product—final dilution.

■ **EXAMPLE 4**

What is the new concentration (% strength) of a dextrose 70% 500 mL solution diluted to 2000 mL?

$Q1 \times C1 = Q2 \times C2$

$500 \text{ mL} \times 70\% = 2000 \text{ mL} \times x\%$

$3500 = 2000x$

$17.5\% = x$

■ **EXAMPLE 5**

How many milliliters of 3% gentamicin solution can be made from 60 mL of 10% gentamicin?

$10\% = \dfrac{10 \text{ g}}{100 \text{ mL}} = \dfrac{x}{60 \text{ mL}} = (10 \text{ g} \times 60 \text{ mL})/100 \text{ mL}$

$\quad = 6 \text{ g gentamicin in 60 mL stock ointment}$

$3\% = \dfrac{3 \text{ g}}{100 \text{ mL}} = \dfrac{6 \text{ g}}{x}$

$x = (6 \text{ g} \times 100 \text{ mL}) \div 3 \text{ g} = 200 \text{ mL}$

Or, try the following formula:

$Q1 \times C1 = Q2 \times C2$

$60 \text{ mL} \times 10\% = x \text{ mL} \times 3\%$

$600 = 3x$

$x = 200 \text{ mL}$

SOLID DILUTIONS

The dilution of solid products (creams and ointments) reduces their concentration also. They can be represented as ratio strengths or percent strengths just like solutions. They are diluted with an ointment or cream base with no active ingredient. The calculations are done the same way as solution dilutions. The proportion rule or quantity/concentration formula can be used.

■ **EXAMPLE 6**

How many grams of lidocaine 20% ointment and how many grams of an ointment base must be combined to obtain 2 lbs of a 2.5% lidocaine topical ointment?

(1 lb = 454 g)

$2.5\% = \dfrac{2.5 \text{ g}}{100 \text{ g}} = \dfrac{x}{908 \text{ g (2 lbs)}}$

$x = (2.5 \text{ g} \times 908 \text{ g}) \div 100 \text{ g} = 22.7 \text{ g lidocaine total in 2 lbs}$

$20\% = \dfrac{20 \text{ g}}{100 \text{ g}} = \dfrac{22.7 \text{ g}}{x}$

$x = (22.7 \text{ g} \times 100 \text{ g}) \div 20 \text{ g} = 113.5 \text{ g}$

113.5 g of lidocaine 20%

794.5 g of ointment base

113.5 + 794.5 = 908 g = 2 lbs

Or, try the following formula:

$Q1 \times C1 = Q2 \times C2$

$x \text{ g} \times 20\% = 908 \text{ g} \times 2.5\%$

$20x = 2270$

$x = 113.5 \text{ g}$ lidocaine 20%

Practice Problems 6.1

1. Sodium acetate 5% solution 100 mL is diluted to a volume of 1000 mL. What is the new percent strength?

2. A solution of 1:400 concentration 250 mL is diluted to 1000 mL. What is the new ratio strength?

3. Niconozole 3% 60 g ointment is combined with 120 g of ointment base. What is the new percent strength?

4. How many milliliters of 4.2% sodium bicarbonate solution can be made from 100 mL of 8.4% concentration?

5. How many grams of betamethasone 0.1% cream can be made from 60 g of a 1% concentration?

6. How many milliliters of a 10% potassium solution are needed to make 180 mL of a 10 mg/mL concentration solution?

7. How much diphenhydramine 2% ointment and how much ointment base are needed to make a 1 lb jar of diphenhydramine 0.5% ointment? (*Hint:* 1 lb = 454 g)

8. How many milliliters of 2% lidocaine are needed to make a 250 mL solution containing 0.4 mg/mL?

9. Hydrocortisone 5% ointment 120 g is added to enough ointment base to make a total volume of 1 lb. What is the new percent strength of hydrocortisone ointment? (*Hint:* 1 lb = 454 g)

10. Cefotaxime comes in 10 g/100 mL concentration. How much diluent must be added to make a concentration of 50 mg/mL?

ALLIGATIONS

Alligations is a method used to calculate the percent strength when combining multiple strengths of the same ingredient. It can also be used when the volume of each of two different strengths of the same ingredient must be determined in order to make a new strength. This new strength must be in-between the two strengths that are being combined.

Alligations medial is the method used to determine the new percent strength when combining multiple strengths of the same ingredient and the volumes are known. There are two different ways to do this calculation.

The first method uses the total volumes of the solutions and the total grams of the ingredient in the solutions, and then, using the proportion rule, the new percent strength is determined.

$$\frac{A \text{ g} + B \text{ g} + C \text{ g}}{A \text{ volume} + B \text{ volume} + C \text{ volume}} = \frac{x \text{ g}}{100 \text{ mL}}$$

$x = \%$ strength

■ **EXAMPLE 7**

Mix together 100 mL of 50% dextrose with 250 mL of 40% dextrose and 450 mL of 70% dextrose. What is the new percent strength?

$50\% = \dfrac{50 \text{ g}}{100 \text{ mL}}$ so 100 mL of 50% solution = 50 g

$40\% = \dfrac{40 \text{ g}}{100 \text{ mL}}$ so 250 mL of 40% solution = 100 g (40×2.5)

$70\% = \dfrac{70 \text{ g}}{100 \text{ mL}}$ so 450 mL of 70% solution = 315 g (70×4.5)

Totals = 800 mL volume   465 g ingredient

$\dfrac{465 \text{ g}}{800 \text{ mL}} = \dfrac{x}{100 \text{ mL}}$

$x = (465 \text{ g} \times 100 \text{ mL}) \div 800 \text{ mL} = 58.125 \text{ g} = 58\%$

The second method uses the percent strengths converted into decimals and then multiplied by their respective volumes. This new volume then is divided by the original volume and the answer is multiplied by 100 to obtain a percent strength.

■ **EXAMPLE 8**

Mix together 100 mL of 50% dextrose with 250 mL of 40% dextrose and 450 mL of 70% dextrose. What is the new percent strength?

$50\% = 0.5 \times 100 \text{ mL} = 50 \text{ mL}$
$40\% = 0.4 \times 250 \text{ mL} = 100 \text{ mL}$
$70\% = 0.7 \times 450 \text{ mL} = 315 \text{ mL}$
Totals: 800 mL 465 mL
465 mL $\div$ 800 mL = $0.58125 \times 100 = 58.125\% = 58\%$

Both methods produce the same answer. As mentioned earlier, the simplest way is not always the best way. Confidence in calculations is important, so the method used (when more than one is possible) depends on the person.

Alligations alternate is the method used to determine the volume necessary for each ingredient combined (i.e., same ingredient, different percent strength) to produce a new percent strength. This new percent strength must be in-between the two being combined.

This method uses a grid to complete the calculations. It resembles a tic-tac-toe board and provides a great visual for calculating. The answers obtained will be the ratio in which the ingredients should be combined. The ratio should always be simplified to it smallest form.

The percent strengths on hand go in the left-hand boxes of the grid, the desired percent strength goes in the middle box, and the "parts" needed are in the right-hand boxes, which translate to the ratio.

The grid should look like this:

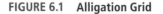

$$\begin{pmatrix} \text{higher\%} & \xrightarrow{\text{parts}} & \text{desired} - \text{lower} \\ \vdots & \text{\% desired} & \vdots \\ \text{lower\%} & \xrightarrow{\text{parts}} & \text{higher} - \text{desired} \end{pmatrix}$$

When the desired strength is subtracted from the higher strength, it represents the parts needed of the lower strength. The lower strength is subtracted from the desired strength (to obtain a positive number), and it represents the parts needed of the higher strength (see **Figure 6.1**).

FIGURE 6.1   Alligation Grid

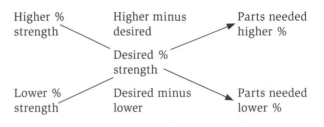

■ **EXAMPLE 9**

A patient needs 70% dextrose and the pharmacy carries 95% and 30% strengths. What proportion is needed to make the 70% solution?

$$\begin{pmatrix} 95 & \rightarrow & 40 \\ & 70 & \\ 30 & \rightarrow & 25 \end{pmatrix}$$ ratio = 40:25, which simplifies to 8:5

(higher %) 95 − (desired %) 70 = 25, which represents the parts needed of lower %
(desired %) 70 − (lower %) 30 = 40, which represents the parts needed of higher %
The ratio of 40:25 can be simplified to 8:5. This means, for every eight parts of 95%, five parts of 30% will be used.

Usually, the volume needed of the new percent strength is known. That information allows the ratio to be further calculated to the exact volume of each solution needed to create the desired percent strength. One step farther would be to know the specific volume of one of the available strengths. That information provides the required volume for the "parts" it represents in the formula.

■ **EXAMPLE 10**

Mix 70% and 30% dextrose to obtain 1000 mL of a 40% concentration.

$$\begin{pmatrix} 70 & \rightarrow & 10 \\ & 40 & \\ 30 & \rightarrow & 30 \end{pmatrix}$$ ratio = 10:30, which simplifies to 1:3

1 part + 3 part = 4 parts total, 1000 mL/4 parts = 250 mL/part
1 part 70% = 250 mL × 1 = 250 mL
3 parts 30% = 250 mL × 3 = $\underline{750 \text{ mL}}$
$\overline{1000 \text{ mL}}$

■ **EXAMPLE 11**

How much 85% aminosyn must be added to 150 mL of 60% aminosyn to make an 80% solution?

$$\begin{pmatrix} 85 & \to & 20 \\ & 80 & \\ 60 & \to & 5 \end{pmatrix} \text{ratio} = 20{:}5, \text{ which simplifies to } 4{:}1$$

The one part represents the 60% aminosyns, which has a known volume of 150 mL. The four parts represent the 85% aminosyn, 150 mL (1 part) × 4 = 600 mL. An 80% solution needs 150 mL of 60% and 600 mL of 85%.

■ **EXAMPLE 12**

Sodium chloride 23.4% and water are mixed to make 2 L of 0.9% sodium chloride.

$$\begin{pmatrix} 234(23.4) & \to & 9 \\ & 9(0.9) & \\ 0 & \to & 225 \end{pmatrix}$$

Remember:
When calculating with decimals, they can be eliminated by moving the decimal point the same number of positions in each number—creating whole numbers. This makes calculating easier.

Water = 0%
Ratio = 9:225, which simplifies to 1:25
Total parts = 1 + 25 = 26 and volume needed is 2000 mL (2 L)
2000 mL/26 = 76.9 mL per part (round to 77 mL)
1 part of 23.4% = 77 mL
25 parts of water (0%) = 76.9 × 25 = 1922.5 mL round to 1923 mL
1923 mL + 77 mL = 2000 mL

Practice Problems 6.2

1. What is the percent strength of a solution containing 400 mL of 50% dextrose, 200 mL of 30% dextrose, and 400 mL of 10% dextrose?

2. How many total grams of aminosyn are in a solution containing 200 mL of 8.5%, 150 mL of 5%, and 50 mL of 10% concentrations?

3. A 70% solution and 20% solution are combined to make a 30% solution. What is the ratio?

4. Dextrose 40% 1000 mL is needed for a patient. The pharmacy only stocks 20% and 50% solutions. How much of each is needed to make the solution?

5. How much 23.4% sodium chloride should be added to 300 mL of sterile water to make a 3% sodium chloride solution? (*Hint:* Remove decimal for calculation—move it to the right one place in both values.)

6. What is the new percent strength when the following zinc oxide ointments are combined?
   (Zinc 10% 60 g, zinc 6% 120 g, zinc 3% 120 g, zinc 5% 150 g)

7. How much 95% dextrose and how much 40% dextrose are needed to obtain a 70% concentration?

8. Potassium chloride 20% 500 mL is ordered. The stock solutions available are 40% and 10%. How much of each is needed to make this solution?

9. How much of each, 20% lidocaine and 30% lidocaine, are needed to make 500 mL of a 28% concentration?

10. Housekeeping needs 1500 mL of a 34% cleansing solution. The stock solutions available are 18% and 42%. How much of each will be used?

CHAPTER 6 QUIZ

1. What is the final concentration (% strength) when you mix 800 g of hydrocortisone 5% cream and 1200 g of hydrocortisone 10% cream?

2. How many grams of dexamethasone 1% ointment can be made from 120 g of dexamethasone 5% ointment?

3. How many milliliters of gentamicin 0.25% ophthalmic solution can be made from a 5 mL stock bottle of gentamicin 2.5% ophthalmic solution?

4. What is the percent strength of epinephrine 1:5000, 1 mL diluted to a volume of 10 mL?

5. A 50% alcohol solution is needed. How many milliliters of sterile water need to be added to 2500 mL of an 83% alcohol solution?

6. Terconazole 8% cream 30 g is diluted to 120 g with cream base. What is the new percent strength?

7. An IV calls for a 500 mL–5% lipid solution. The stock solution available is 20%. How many milliliters of 20% lipids and how many milliliters of sterile water are needed for this IV?

8. A patient needs 50 mL of a 5% dextrose solution. How many milliliters of 70% dextrose and how many milliliters of water will be needed to make this solution?

9. A stock bottle of calcium gluconate has concentration of 10 mg/mL. The prescription calls for 10 mL of a 4 mg/mL concentration. How many milliliters of calcium gluconate and how many milliliters of water are needed to fill this prescription?

10. Folic acid 50 mcg/mL, 30 mL is ordered. The stock vial is 5 mg/mL. How many milliliters of folic acid and how many milliliters of sterile water must be combined to fill this order?

11. An IV of dextrose 12.5% 500 mL is ordered. The pharmacy only stocks D10%W and D20%W. How many milliliters of each will be needed?

12. Dextrose 8% 400 mL is ordered. Make this solution from D20% and sterile water. How many milliliters of each solution will be needed?

13. Sodium chloride 0.45% 500 mL is ordered. Make this solution from 23.4% sodium chloride and sterile water. How many milliliters of each will be needed? (*Hint:* Eliminate decimals for an easier calculation.)

14. Triamcinolone cream 3% 60 g is needed. The stock available is a 10% cream and a 1% cream. How many grams of each will be used?

15. Isoproterenol 1:400 20 mL is combined with isoproterenol 1:150 80 mL. What is the new concentration in ratio strength? In percent strength?

16. Metronidazole cream 2% 30 g is mixed with metronidazole cream 8% 30 g. What is the new percent strength?

17. Mix together dextrose 15% 1000 mL, dextrose 3% 500 mL, dextrose 70% 300 mL, and dextrose 40% 200 mL. What is the new percent concentration?

18. Mix together alcohol 50% 100 mL, alcohol 95% 100 mL, and alcohol 70% 100 mL. What is the new percent concentration?

19. Combine betamethasone 0.1% ointment 60 g, betamethasone 1% ointment 60 g, and betamethasone 3% ointment 120 g. What is the new percent strength?

20. Prepare 4 L of 28% iodine solution. The stock solutions available are 16% and 32%. How many milliliters of each solution are needed?

Dosing

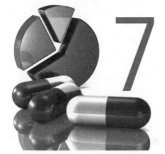

OBJECTIVES

- Be able to define geriatric dosing guidelines
- Be able to calculate geriatric doses
- Be able to define pediatric dosing guidelines
- Be able to calculate pediatric doses
- Be able to calculate chemotherapy doses

GERIATRICS

Geriatric patients are generally classified as persons over 60 years of age. This is relative because some patients may have geriatric symptoms at 50 years of age or even younger. As we age, our physiologic functions start to decline. Kidney function and liver function are two major concerns when dosing medications in elderly patients. These both affect the absorption and elimination of medications. When medications remain in the body longer, they accumulate in the blood and tissues creating increased drug levels, which cause toxicity.

Drugs are often dosed using body surface area (BSA). Some medications have guidelines for reduced dosing based on the patients weight and age. Renal (kidney) function can also play a role in dosing a medication. If the kidneys are not functioning properly, reduced doses are often prescribed. Creatinine clearance is the lab value physicians and pharmacists use to determine kidney function and appropriate dosing for elderly patients. Medications will have dosing guidelines for reduced kidney function to prevent toxicity.

BSA is the calculation we focus on in this book. It is used for geriatric, pediatric, and chemotherapy dosing. The formula is the same for all three applications. There is a preprinted nomogram that can be used to determine a patient's BSA by knowing his or her height and weight. Many reference books have this chart included. Most pharmacy computer programs have this calculation in its formula banks, which eliminates manual calculating and potential error.

The formula is slightly different depending on the information format. There is a formula for inches and pounds and a formula for centimeters and kilograms. Both are height and weight measures; one in apothecary and one in metric.

$$\text{BSA} \rightarrow \text{m}^2 \sqrt{\frac{\text{height (cm)} \times \text{weight (kg)}}{3600}}$$

$$\text{BSA} \rightarrow \text{m}^2 \sqrt{\frac{\text{height (in.)} \times \text{weight (lbs)}}{3131}}$$

▪ EXAMPLE 1

A gentleman weighs 110 kg and is 180 cm tall. What is his BSA?

$$\sqrt{\frac{180 \text{ cm} \times 110 \text{ kg}}{3600}} = \sqrt{\frac{19,800}{3600}} = \sqrt{5.5} = 2.34 \text{ m}^2$$

▪ EXAMPLE 2

A patient weighs 150 lbs and is 65 in. tall. What is the BSA?

$$\sqrt{\frac{65 \text{ in.} \times 150 \text{ lbs}}{3131}} = \sqrt{\frac{9750}{3131}} = \sqrt{3.114} = 1.76 \text{ m}^2$$

PEDIATRICS

Pediatric patients are classified as persons under the age of 18 (see **Table 7.1**). They should be dosed based on their weight or BSA. Accuracy in dosing pediatric patients is very important. Toxicity can occur at much smaller doses. There are several formulas that can be used if the BSA is not known or if the drug does not require a BSA to determine the dose. While age does play a role, weight is still the best way to dose when the BSA is not known. When dosing by weight, the drug product tells you the dosing guidelines (50 mg/kg/dose).

There are three formulas commonly used to determine a child's dose using the known adult dose. **Young's Rule** uses the age of the patient and the adult dose. **Fried's Rule** is for infants and uses the age (in months) of the infant and the adult dose. **Clark's Rule** uses the weight of the patient and the adult dose.

Young's Rule:

$$\frac{\text{Age}}{\text{Age} + 12} \times \text{Adult dose} = \text{Child's dose}$$

TABLE 7.1   Age Breakdown of Pediatric Patients

Name	Age
Neonatal	Birth–1 month
Infant	1 month–2 yrs
Child	2 yrs–12 yrs
Adolescent	13 yrs–17 yrs

Fried's Rule:

$$\frac{\text{Age (next birthday)} \times \text{Adult dose}}{12} = \text{Child's dose}$$

Clark's Rule:

$$\frac{\text{Weight (lbs)} \times \text{Adult dose}}{150} = \text{Child's dose}$$

■ EXAMPLE 3

A 6-year-old child weighs 42 lbs. The adult dose of antibiotic is 375 mg. What is the child's dose? (The package insert doses at 5 mg/kg/dose.)

1. Weight: 42 lbs ÷ 2.2 kg = 19 kg

    19 kg × 5 mg = 95 mg

2. Young's Rule: $\dfrac{6}{6+12} \times 375 \text{ mg} = 125 \text{ mg}$

3. Clark's Rule: $\dfrac{42 \times 375 \text{ mg}}{150} = 105 \text{ mg}$

There is a 10% dose difference in the weight calculation versus Clark's calculation and a 30% dose difference versus Young's calculation. The general rule for margin of error in dosing is 5% or less. Since weight dosing is the most accurate of the three, the others might very well overdose the patient. Age is the biggest variable when it comes to dosing. A child who is 6 years old and weighs 42 lbs should be dosed much differently than a 6-year-old who weighs 65 lbs.

Practice Problems 7.1

Calculate the BSA.

1. Patient weighs 40 lbs and is 42 in. tall.
2. Patient weighs 220 lbs and is 72 in. tall.
3. Patient weighs 80 kg and is 175 cm tall.
4. Patient weighs 2 kg and is 41 cm tall.

Calculate the following doses.

5. Amikacin 5 mg/kg/dose and patient weighs 80 kg.
6. Amoxicillin 10 mg/kg/dose and patient weighs 33 lbs.
7. Ranitidine 2.5 mg/kg/dose and patient weighs 176 lbs.
8. Ticarcillin 200 mg/kg/day and patient weighs 25 kg.
9. A patient weighing 55 lbs has an order for clindamycin every 8 hr. Clindamycin is dosed at 15 mg/kg/day. How much is each dose?

Calculate the following doses using Young's Rule and Clark's Rule.

10. Ibuprofen is ordered for a 5-year-old child weighing 40 lbs. The adult dose is 600 mg.
11. Metronidazole is ordered for an 8-year-old child weighing 65 lbs. The adult dose is 500 mg.
12. Diphenhydramine is ordered for a 2-year-old child weighing 20 lbs. The adult dose is 50 mg.

13. Erythromycin is ordered for a 6-year-old child weighing 50 lbs. The adult dose is 1 g (1000 mg).

14. Metoclopramide is ordered for an 11-year-old child weighing 80 lbs. The adult dose is 10 mg.

CHEMOTHERAPY

Chemotherapy agents are medications that are used for cancer. They are very potent, hazardous chemicals that cause cell death. Because these agents are so hazardous, dosing them correctly is critical. These medications are normally dosed based on BSA and take into consideration kidney (renal) function.

The measure of kidney function is the serum creatinine lab value. This value is then used in a formula to determine the patient's creatinine clearance that is then used to determine dosing of certain medications. Creatinine is a product of creatine phosphate from muscle metabolism. The normal value for serum creatinine used by most laboratories is 0.7–1.5 mg/dL. If this value is above 1.5, the patient has decreased renal function. Decreased renal function means the medication dose must be reduced. Likewise, if the creatinine is lower than 0.7, the patient has increased renal function. The medication may need to be dosed higher so the medication can remain in the body long enough to elicit a therapeutic effect.

While technicians do not do this calculation often, it is good to know how and where the values are used. Pharmacy computer programs usually have this calculation in their system, but when computers fail, knowing how to determine creatinine clearance manually can allow patient dosing to continue.

Manufacturers of these hazardous medications provide detailed dosing information regarding BSA, renal function, and many other lab values that might create the need to alter a dose for a patient. They may suggest a specific dose or a percent reduction of a standard dose.

The formula for creatinine clearance in a male patient is:

$$CrCl = \frac{(140 - age) \times weight\ (kg)}{72 \times serum\ Cr}$$

The formula for a female patient is:

$$CrCl = 0.85 \times \frac{(140 - age) \times weight\ (kg)}{72 \times serum\ Cr}$$

The numbers 140 and 72 are constants in the formula. The serum Cr (serum creatinine) value is obtained from the lab. The weight of the patient must be converted to kilograms. The 0.85 is an adjustment factor for female patients.

■ **EXAMPLE 4**

Patient is 62 years old and weighs 154 lbs. Serum creatinine is 1.9 mg/dL.

Male: $CrCl = \dfrac{(140 - 62) \times 70\ kg}{72 \times 1.9\ mg/dL} = \dfrac{5460}{136.8} = 39.91\ mL/min$

Female: $CrCl = 0.85 \times \dfrac{(140 - 62) \times 70\ kg}{72 \times 1.9\ mg/dL} = 0.85 \times \dfrac{5460}{136.8} = 33.93\ mL/min$

Practice Problems 7.2

Calculate the creatinine clearance.

1. Patient is a 65-year-old male and weighs 175 lbs. The serum creatinine is 1.9 mg/dL.
2. Patient is a 42-year-old female and weighs 140 lbs. The serum creatinine is 1.2 mg/dL.
3. Patient is an 84-year-old male and weighs 160 lbs. The serum creatinine is 2.1 mg/dL.
4. Patient is a 75-year-old female and weighs 155 lbs. The serum creatinine is 1.8 mg/dL.
5. Patient is a 90-year-old female and weighs 110 lbs. The serum creatinine is 2.0 mg/dL.

Calculate the dose based on BSA and CrCl.

Cyclophosphamide 500 mg/m²

Reduce dose by 10% CrCl < 35 mL/min

Reduce dose by 25% CrCl < 20 mL/min

6. Patient is a 75-year-old male, weighs 165 lbs, and is 67 in. tall with serum creatinine 1.8 mg/dL.
7. Patient is 62-year-old female, weighs 121 lbs, and is 65 in. tall with serum creatinine 1.7 mg/dL.

CHAPTER 7 QUIZ

Calculate the BSA. Remember to use the correct formula.

1. Patient is 60 in. tall and weighs 75 kg.
2. Patient is 165 cm tall and weighs 70 kg.
3. Patient is 70 in. tall and weighs 200 lbs.
4. Patient is 30 in. tall and weighs 32 lbs.
5. Patient is 70 cm tall and weighs 20 lbs.

Calculate the dose.

1. Medication is dosed at 12 mg/kg/day. The patient weighs 187 lbs.
2. Cefazolin is ordered 75 mg/kg/day divided into three doses. The patient weighs 25 kg. How much is needed for one dose?
3. Gentamicin 1.75 mg/kg/dose. Patient weighs 132 lbs.
4. Hydrocortisone 0.5 mg/kg/dose. Patient weighs 60 kg.
5. Ibuprofen 20 mg/kg/day. Patient weighs 275 lbs.

Calculate dose using BSA.

1. Paclitaxol is ordered at 135 mg/m². Patient weighs 132 lbs and is 66 in. tall.
2. Vincristine is ordered at 2 mg/m². Patient weighs 55 kg and is 167 cm tall.
3. Amikacin is ordered at 100 mg/m². Patient weighs 22 lbs and is 26 in. tall.

4. Carboplatin is ordered at 150 mg/m². Patient weighs 220 lbs and is 72 in. tall.
5. Methotrexate is ordered at 25 mg/m². Patient weighs 165 lbs and is 69 in. tall.

Calculate creatinine clearance.

1. Patient weighs 82 kg and is a 70-year-old male. Serum creatinine is 1.9 mg/dL.
2. Patient is a 65-year-old female who weighs 150 lbs. Serum creatinine is 1.8 mg/dL.
3. Patient is a 45-year-old female who weighs 135 lbs. Serum creatinine is 1.6 mg/dL.
4. Patient weighs 65 kg and is a 92-year-old male. Serum creatinine is 2.1 mg/dL.
5. Patient weighs 125 kg and is a 54-year-old male. Serum creatinine is 1.7 mg/dL.

Calculate the dose. Use the information provided to determine which formula is needed.

1. A patient weighs 12 kg. Acetaminophen w/codeine is ordered at 0.5 mg/kg/dose.
2. A patient has a BSA of 0.82 m². Gangcyclovir 250 mg/m² is ordered.
3. Mitomycin 25 mg/m² is ordered. Patient weighs 185 lbs and is 71 in. tall.
4. Acyclovir 250 mg/m² is ordered. Patient weighs 22 lbs and is 30 in. tall.
5. Ampicillin 40 mg/kg/day is ordered. Patient weighs 12 kg and is 2 years old.
6. Erythromycin 50 mg/kg/day is ordered. Patient weighs 132 lbs and is 20 years old.
7. Child is 8 years old. The adult dose of medication is 750 mg.
8. Child is 32 lbs. The adult dose of medication is 150 mg.
9. Levothyroxine 5 mcg/kg is ordered. The patient weighs 95 kg.
10. Cisplatin 150 mg/m² is ordered. The patient is a 58-year-old male, weighs 209 lbs, and is 69 in. tall. The serum creatinine is 1.8 mg/dL. The physician ordered a 10% dose reduction.
    a. What is the BSA?
    b. What is the CrCl?
    c. What is the calculated dose?
    d. What is the reduced dose?

IV Admixture Calculations

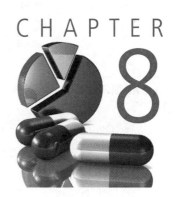

OBJECTIVES

- Be able to calculate the amount of drug to be added to an IV solution
- Be able to calculate drug additive volumes for TPN solutions
- Be able to calculate IV flow rates
- Be able to calculate the length of time of an IV infusion

INTRAVENOUS MEDICATIONS

An intravenous (IV) medication is a drug that is in a liquid, or liquid-like, state that is administered with a syringe and needle. It may be given just under the skin (subcutaneous [SQ]), directly into a muscle (intramuscular [IM]), directly into a vein (intravenous push [IVP]), or slowly infused into the vein through dilution in an IV fluid (parenteral IV infusion). Many of these medications come in bulk packaging, which requires either dilution, or simple calculations to determine the volume needed for a patient dose. Most medications are dosed in milligrams or grams. These are common measures and have been utilized throughout this text. There are two other measures seen in IV medications: milliequivalents (mEq) and units.

MILLIEQUIVALENTS

The milliequivalent is most often used in electrolyte solutions. Calcium, sodium, potassium, chloride, sulfate, and phosphates are the common ones used in pharmacies. The milliequivalent is a measure of the ratio between a molecule's weight and its valence electrons. For calculating purposes, it is treated no differently than a medication measured in milligrams or grams. The notation of dosage strength (mEq/mL) is the only difference. Potassium chloride comes in 2 mEq/mL concentration while ferrous sulfate comes in 300 mg/5 mL, or 60 mg/mL concentration. A physician will order the appropriate dose for the medication desired.

An oral dose of a medication is ordered for a specific quantity over a specific period of time—ampicillin 500 mg four times a day for 10 days. An IV medication may be ordered based on the volume of a solution it will be added to and run over a specific amount of time—potassium chloride 30 mEq/1000 mL to be run over 8 hr. If the patient already has a bag of solution hanging and it has less than 1000 mL in it, then the dose must be adjusted according to the remaining volume.

■ **EXAMPLE 1**

A physician orders sodium chloride 40 mEq/1000 mL. The patient has 400 mL remaining in the current bag. How much needs to be added? The pharmacy stock is 4 mEq/mL.

$$\frac{40 \text{ mEq}}{1000 \text{ mL}} = \frac{x}{400 \text{ mL}}$$

$x = (40 \text{ mEq} \times 400 \text{ mL}) \div 1000 \text{ mL} = 16 \text{ mEq needed}$

$$\frac{16 \text{ mEq}}{x} = \frac{4 \text{ mEq}}{1 \text{ mL}}$$

$x = 4 \text{ mL}$

UNITS

The unit is a measurement used in insulin, some vitamins, heparin, penicillin, some blood products, and various other medications. The unit is a measure of a particular medication's activity based on a test system for that specific agent. These test systems are biological assays designed to define a specific medication's "unit" of activity. A unit of insulin is not measured the same as a unit of heparin or a unit of vitamin E. Insulin is based on its affect on glucose in the bloodstream. Heparin is based on its anticoagulation effect in the bloodstream.

Insulin is measured by its units with syringes available that are designed specifically for measuring insulin doses. The standard concentration of insulin is 100 units per 1 mL or 100 units/mL. Physicians order insulin by the unit based on the patient's blood glucose level. They may have multiple doses ordered—10 units before breakfast, 20 units before dinner.

■ **EXAMPLE 2**

A patient needs insulin 15 units, SQ, at breakfast and 20 units, SQ, at dinner. How much insulin is needed for each dose? Insulin is available in 100 units/mL concentration.

$$\frac{15 \text{ units}}{x} = \frac{100 \text{ units}}{1 \text{ mL}} \qquad\qquad \frac{20 \text{ units}}{x} = \frac{100 \text{ units}}{1 \text{ mL}}$$

$x = 0.15 \text{ mL}$ $\qquad\qquad\qquad\qquad x = 0.2 \text{ mL}$

■ **EXAMPLE 3**

A physician ordered 36 units of regular insulin to be added to a patient's IV. Regular insulin is 100 units/mL.

$$\frac{100 \text{ units}}{1 \text{ mL}} = \frac{36 \text{ units}}{x}$$

$x = 0.36 \text{ mL}$

Heparin is ordered in units also. It can be administered SQ or as an IV infusion. Heparin comes in a variety of concentrations, unlike insulin. Heparin is available in 10 units/mL, 100 units/mL, 1000 units/mL, 5000 units/mL, and 10,000 units/mL. The concentration used depends on the dose desired and route of administration. If a patient needs 10,000 units of heparin SQ, the 5000 unit/mL concentration is not a good choice. A SQ dose should be 1 mL or less because it is given just under the skin. If the 10,000 units of heparin are to be added to an IV infusion, it does not matter which concentration is used because it is being further diluted and administered through the patient's veins.

■ **EXAMPLE 4**

Heparin 7500 units SQ is ordered for a patient. The pharmacy carries 5000 units/mL and 10,000 units/mL. Which strength should be used? How much is needed for the dose?

$$\frac{7500 \text{ units}}{x} = \frac{5000 \text{ units}}{1 \text{ mL}} \qquad\qquad \frac{7500 \text{ units}}{x} = \frac{10,000 \text{ units}}{1 \text{ mL}}$$

$$x = 1.5 \text{ mL} \qquad\qquad\qquad\qquad x = 0.75 \text{ mL}$$

The 5000 units/mL has a volume greater than 1 mL, which is not appropriate for a SQ dose. The 10,000 units/mL has a volume less than 1 mL, which is the best choice for the desired dose.

Practice Problems 8.1

1. A physician ordered 15 mEq of potassium chloride in normal saline (NS) 100 mL. How much potassium chloride will be added to the NS? Potassium chloride is available as 2 mEq/mL.

2. Potassium phosphate 60 mEq/1000 mL is ordered. The patient has 750 mL remaining in the current IV bag. How much should be added to this current IV bag? Potassium phosphate is available as 4.4 mEq/mL.

3. An order for regular insulin calls for 12 units/100 mL. The patient has a 500 mL bag of NS currently hanging. How many units of insulin must be added? How many milliliters of insulin are needed for the dose? Insulin is available as 100 units/mL.

4. Penicillin 5 million units in NS 100 mL every 4 hrs is ordered. How many milliliters are needed for one dose? Penicillin is available as 500,000 units/mL.

5. Heparin 25,000 units/250 mL is ordered. The patient has 200 mL remaining in the IV bag. How much heparin should be added to the patient's IV bag? The heparin available is 10,000 units/mL.

TPN SOLUTIONS

Total parenteral solution (TPN) is an IV that provides nutrition to patients who cannot eat normally. They have multiple additives that are customized to the patient's nutritional needs. These IVs have a dextrose solution and an amino acid solution as the base that represents the sugar (carbohydrate) and proteins portions of a traditional diet. Additives often include potassium, sodium, calcium, and multivitamins. They can also include insulin, trace elements, heparin, and an H_2 antagonist (reduces the production of stomach acid). The quantities of each additive are determined by lab values that are drawn daily in the beginning and then weekly if the patient is on TPN therapy for a length of time.

■ **EXAMPLE 5**

TPN Order:

Amino acids 8.5% 500 mL
Dextrose 50% 500 mL
Potassium chloride (KCl) 40 mEq   *(stock solution = 2 mEq/mL)*
Sodium chloride (NaCl) 24 mEq   *(stock solution = 4 mEq/mL)*
Calcium gluconate 1 g   *(stock solution = 1 g/10 mL)*
Insulin 24 units   *(stock solution = 100 units/mL)*

How much of each additive is needed for this TPN?

$$KCl \frac{40 \text{ mEq}}{x} = \frac{2 \text{ mEq}}{1 \text{ mL}}$$

$$x = 20 \text{ mL}$$

$$CaGluc \frac{1 \text{ g}}{10 \text{ mL}} = 10 \text{ mL}$$

$$NaCl \frac{24 \text{ mEq}}{x} = \frac{4 \text{ mEq}}{1 \text{ mL}}$$

$$x = 6 \text{ mL}$$

$$Insulin \frac{24 \text{ units}}{x} = \frac{100 \text{ units}}{1 \text{ mL}}$$

$$x = 0.24 \text{ mL}$$

Sometimes the additives will be ordered based on a volume: 40 mEq/1000 mL. Many TPN orders are written for a 24-hr period. If the final volume of the TPN solution is 2500 mL, then the additives are calculated on that desired final volume.

■ **EXAMPLE 6**

TPN Order:

Amino acids 10% 1000 mL
Dextrose 40% 1000 mL
Lipids 10% 500 mL
KCl 30 mEq/1000 mL   *(stock = 2 mEq/mL)*
Sodium acetate 20 mEq/1000 mL   *(stock = 4 mEq/mL)*
Potassium phosphate 15 mEq/1000 mL   *(stock = 4.4 mEq/mL)*
Insulin 8 units/1000 mL   *(stock = 100 units/mL)*

Total volume of TPN base solutions = 2500 mL

$$KCl \frac{30 \text{ mEq}}{1000 \text{ mL}} = \frac{x}{2500 \text{ mL}}$$

$$x = 75 \text{ mEq}$$

$$\frac{75 \text{ mEq}}{x} = \frac{2 \text{ mEq}}{1 \text{ mL}}$$

$$x = 37.5 \text{ mL}$$

SodAcetate $\dfrac{20 \text{ mEq}}{1000 \text{ mL}} = \dfrac{x}{2500 \text{ mL}}$ $\dfrac{50 \text{ mEq}}{x} = \dfrac{4 \text{ mEq}}{1 \text{ mL}}$

$x = 50 \text{ mEq}$ $x = 12.5 \text{ mL}$

KPhos $\dfrac{15 \text{ mEq}}{1000 \text{ mL}} = \dfrac{x}{2500 \text{ mL}}$ $\dfrac{37.5 \text{ mEq}}{x} = \dfrac{4.4 \text{ mEq}}{1 \text{ mL}}$

$x = 37.5 \text{ mEq}$ $x = 8.5 \text{ mL}$

Insulin $\dfrac{8 \text{ units}}{1000 \text{ mL}} = \dfrac{x}{2500 \text{ mL}}$ $\dfrac{20 \text{ units}}{x} = \dfrac{100 \text{ units}}{1 \text{ mL}}$

$x = 20 \text{ units}$ $x = 0.2 \text{ mL}$

IV FLOW RATES

When IV solutions are ordered they must have a rate of administration. It might be run over a specific time—20 min, or at a continual rate—100 mL/hr. A general rule is that an IV solution with 250 mL or less is considered a "piggyback" and infused through a main IV line over a set period of time. Large volumes are considered 500 mL or more and are run at a continual rate.

Knowing the rate of administration will help the technician determine how many IV bags need to be prepared for a patient. Most hospital pharmacies prepare IVs for a 24-hr period. If an IV is running at 125 mL/hr and the order is for 1000 mL, then the patient needs three bags—1000 mL ÷ 125 mL = 8 hrs; 24 hrs ÷ 8 hrs = 3 bags.

■ **EXAMPLE 7**

An IV of 1000 mL is running at 100 mL/hr. How many hours will it last? How many bags are needed for a 24-hr period?

$\dfrac{1000 \text{ mL}}{100 \text{ mL}} = 10 \text{ hr}; \quad 24 \text{ hr} \div 10 \text{ hr} = 2.4 \text{ bags}$

■ **EXAMPLE 8**

A 500 mL IV bag needs to run over 6 hr. What is the rate of administration?

$\dfrac{500 \text{ mL}}{6 \text{ hr}} = 83.3 \text{ mL/hr}$

Some IV orders are written with an administration rate of mL/min instead of mL/hr. This calculation simply replaces the hours with minutes (1 hr = 60 min).

■ **EXAMPLE 9**

An IV bag of 1 L is running at 75 mL/hr. What is the rate in mL/min?

$$\frac{75 \text{ mL}}{60 \text{ min (1 hr)}} = \frac{x}{\text{min}}$$

$$x = 1.25 \text{ mL/min}$$

DROP SETS

IV solutions are administered using IV tubing sets. These sets are called drip sets, drop sets, or microdrip sets. Each one delivers a set number of drops in 1 mL. This information can be used to determine the rate at which an IV is administered. While nursing generally performs these calculations, pharmacy staff should be able to assist as a double check. The most common sets have a drip rate of 10, 15, 20, and 60 drops per milliliter (gtts/mL). The 60 gtts/mL tubing is often called a microdrip set. To convert a rate from mL/hr to gtts/min, the following formula can be used:

$$\text{gtts/min} = \frac{(\text{volume/hr}) \times \text{drop rate}}{60 \text{ min/hr}}$$

■ **EXAMPLE 10**

An IV is being administered at 75 mL/hr. What is the gtts/min for a 20 gtt/mL tubing?

$$\text{gtts/min} = \frac{(75 \text{ mL/hr}) \times 20 \text{ gtts/mL}}{60 \text{ min/hr}} = \frac{1500}{60} = 25 \text{ gtts/min}$$

Nursing staff can use this information to calibrate an IV tubing manually. There are still some IVs that are not required to run on a pump, so the rate must be set by counting the drops per minute.

Sometimes the mL/hr rate is not given. The order may ask for a specific volume to be delivered over a set time. By knowing the drop rate of the tubing being used, the gtts/min can be calculated. This can then be used to calibrate the drip rate of the tubing to deliver the medication in the time requested by the physician.

■ **EXAMPLE 11**

Cefazolin 1 g in 50 mL NS is to run over 20 min. The nursing staff chooses a 15 gtts/mL tubing. What is the rate in gtts/min? *Hint*: 20 min = $\frac{1}{3}$ (0.3) of an hour.

$$\text{gtts/min} = \frac{(50 \text{ mL/0.3}) \times 15 \text{ gtts/mL}}{60 \text{ min/hr}} = \frac{2500}{60} = 41.67 \text{ gtts/min}$$

The amount of drug being delivered or the total volume delivered can be calculated when the gtts/min is known. This information is useful when a physician orders a medication to be administered in gtts/min. The pharmacy can then determine how much drug should be used or the volume of solution needed to run over a set time (e.g., 1 hr, 6 hr).

■ **EXAMPLE 12**

An IV is running at 30 gtts/min through a 10 gtts/mL tubing. How many milliliters will be needed for 24 hr?

1. mL/min $\dfrac{30 \text{ gtts}}{1 \text{ min}} \times \dfrac{1 \text{ mL}}{10 \text{ gtts}} = 3 \text{ mL/min}$

2. mL/hr $\dfrac{3 \text{ mL}}{\text{min}} = \dfrac{1 \text{ hr}}{60 \text{ min}} = 180 \text{ mL/hr}$

3. 180 mL × 24 hr = 4320 mL = 4.32 L

Practice Problems 8.2

1. A patient has an IV order for lactated ringers (LR) 1500 mL at 80 mL/hr. What is the rate in gtts/min if the nurse uses a 60 gtts/mL set?

2. An IV is running at 100 mL/hr. How many 1000 mL bags are needed for a 24-hr period?

3. What is the gtts/min rate for a 50 mL bag of cimetidine if it is to run over 30 min using a 20 gtts/mL tubing?

4. Lidocaine 0.4% 500 mL is ordered to run at 30 gtts/min. How long will the bag last if a 15 gtts/mL tubing is used?

5. Dextrose 5% 1000 mL will last for 12 hr. What is the rate in mL/hr?

6. TPN Order:

   Dextrose 20% 500 mL

   Amino acids 5% 500 mL

KCl 60 mEq	*(stock = 2 mEq/mL)*
NaCl 40 mEq	*(stock = 4 mEq/mL)*
CaGluc 750 mg	*(stock = 1 g/10 mL)*
KPhos 15 mEq	*(stock = 4.4 mEq/mL)*
Insulin 16 units	*(stock = 100 units/mL)*

   Base solution volume = 1000 mL

   Run this IV over 8 hr

   a. How much is needed of each additive for this TPN?

   b. What is the rate in mL/hr?

   c. What is the rate in gtts/min for a 60 gtts/mL tubing?

CHAPTER 8 QUIZ

1. Heparin 20,000 units/mL is available. How many units are in 0.6 mL?

2. Penicillin G 4.5 million units is ordered for a patient. The pharmacy stocks a 500,000 units/mL solution. How many milliliters are needed for this order?

3. D5 $\frac{1}{2}$ NS 1000 mL w/40 mEq KCl is ordered. How much potassium is needed if the pharmacy carries a 2 mEq/mL concentration?

4. NaCl 60 mEq/1000 mL is ordered. The patient has only 800 mL remaining in the IV bag. How much NaCl must be added if the stock solution is 4 mEq/mL?

5. Vitamin E 400 units are ordered. The pharmacy stocks 1000 units/5 mL. How much is needed for this dose?

6. LR 1000 mL will run from 7 AM to 3 PM.

   a. What is the rate in mL/hr?
   b. How much is remaining after 5 hr?
   c. What is the rate in gtts/min for a 15 gtts/mL tubing?

7. NS 500 mL runs for 24 hr. What is the rate in mL/hr?

8. TPN Order:

   Dextrose 70% 1000 mL

   Amino acids 8.5% 1000 mL

   Lipids 20% 500 mL

   NaCl 30 mEq/1000 mL   *(stock = 4 mEq/mL)*

   KCl 15 mEq/1000 mL   *(stock = 2 mEq/mL)*

   Cimetidine 150 mg/1000 mL   *(stock = 300 mg/2 mL)*

   Insulin 5 units/1000 mL   *(stock = 100 units/mL)*

   Base solution volume = 2500 mL

   Run over 24 hr

   a. How much of each additive is needed?
   b. What is the rate in mL/hr?
   c. What is the rate in gtts/min for a 20 gtts/mL tubing?

9. Vancomycin 750 mg in NS 250 mL is run over 90 min. What is the gtts/min for a 20 gtts/mL tubing?

10. How long will a 1000 mL bag of D5LR last if it is running at 40 gtts/min through a 20 gtts/mL tubing?

Business Math

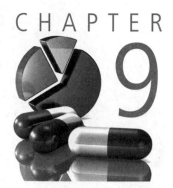

OBJECTIVES

- Define average wholesale price
- Calculate selling price
- Calculate net profit
- Calculate gross profit
- Calculate insurance reimbursement
- Define markup and add-on fees
- Calculate inventory turnover

INVENTORY

All saleable items found in a pharmacy are considered inventory. Inventory is one of the largest costs in a pharmacy. Pharmacies want to turn over their inventory as often as possible. If an item sits on a shelf, it is costing the pharmacy money. The turnover rate is the total number of times the pharmacy's inventory has been replaced in one year:

Turnover rate = annual inventory purchased ÷ average inventory

The annual inventory is the sum of the year's invoices. The average inventory is the value of the inventory maintained on a daily basis. If the annual invoices total $100,000 and the average inventory is $20,000, then the turnover rate is five (100,000 ÷ 20,000). A good turnover rate is four or more.

■ **EXAMPLE 1**

A pharmacy maintains an average inventory of $32,000. The annual purchases total $200,000. What is the turnover rate?

$$\text{Turnover} = \frac{200,000}{32,000} = 6.25 \text{ turns}$$

PROFIT

The amount of money made on the sale of an item is the profit. The two types of profit are gross profit and net profit. The gross profit is the difference in the selling price and the purchase price. The net profit is the selling price minus all costs associated with the dispensing of the product. These costs might include pharmacy supplies (e.g., labels, bottles), personnel time, and shipping fees.

■ EXAMPLE 2

Propranolol 40 mg #100 costs the pharmacy $14.50. The prescription price is $42.00. What is the gross profit?

Gross profit = $42.00 − $14.50 = $27.50

■ EXAMPLE 3

Propranolol 40 mg #100 costs the pharmacy $14.50. Dispensing costs for this prescription total $12.40. The prescription price is $42.00. What is the net profit?

Net profit = $42.00 − $14.50 − $12.40 = $15.10

Practice Problems 9.1

1. The annual purchases for Pharmacy A totals $750,000. The average inventory is $192,000. What is the turnover rate?
2. A prescription sells for $56. The medication cost is $22 and dispensing costs are $13. What is the gross profit? What is the net profit?
3. A prescription sells for $110. The medication cost is $72 and dispensing costs are $22. What is the gross profit? What is the net profit?
4. The pharmacy had annual purchases of $250,000. The average inventory is $100,000. What is the turnover rate?
5. A prescription sells for $18. The medication cost is $4 and dispensing costs are $7.50. What is the gross profit? What is the net profit?

SELLING PRICE

The selling price of a prescription is based on several factors. The pharmacy must charge enough to cover the cost of the drug, the cost of acquiring the drug, and the time invested in dispensing the drug. The average wholesale price (AWP) is used to determine the selling price of medications. The AWP is the average price charged by wholesalers for that product. Most wholesalers offer a discount based on volume or contracting with large chains.

■ EXAMPLE 4

Wholesaler A offers an 8% discount on imipramine 25 mg if 10 or more are purchased. The AWP is $53. Joe's Pharmacy orders 12 bottles. How much did they pay per bottle?

$53.00 × 0.08 = $4.24
$53.00 − $4.24 = $48.76 per bottle

Pharmacies add a markup percent or flat rate and sometimes a dispensing fee, compounding fee, or professional fee to the cost they pay for a medication to determine the selling price. The markup percent or flat rate is set by the individual pharmacy or pharmacy chain. Sometimes the percent or flat rate is tiered based on the cost of the drug. The compounding fee and professional fee are based on time or a flat rate.

■ EXAMPLE 5

Joe's Pharmacy has a markup rate of 15% and charges a $5 dispensing fee. How much is a prescription for digoxin 0.125 mg, 100 tablets if Joe's cost was $32?

$32.00 + (32 × 0.15) + $5.00 = $32.00 + $4.80 + $5.00 = $41.80

■ EXAMPLE 6

Joe's Pharmacy also charges a compounding fee when they have to fill a prescription that must be mixed or made from a recipe. The compounding fee is $60 per hour.

Bacitracin ointment 15 g	*$4.50*
Zinc oxide 15 g	*$3.00*
Camphor 10 mL	*$2.00*

How much will this prescription cost if it took 20 min to compound? (Remember to include the markup and dispensing fee from Example 5.)

$4.50 + $3.00 + $2.00 = $9.50 of ingredients
$9.50 + (9.50 × 0.15) + $5.00 = $9.50 + 1.43 + $5.00 = $15.93
$15.93 + compounding fee (20 min) = $15.93 + (60.00 ÷ 3) = $35.93

■ EXAMPLE 7

Joe's Pharmacy dispenses a prescription for citalopram 20 mg #40. The cost for 100 tablets is $260. (Remember to include the dispensing and markup fees from Example 5.)

$260.00/100 tablets = $2.60 per tablet × 40 tablets = $104.00 cost for 40 tablets
$104.00 + (104 × 0.15) + $5.00 = $104.00 + $15.60 + $5.00 = $124.60

When calculating prescription pricing, remember the following guidelines:

1. Determine the cost per unit (e.g., tablet, ounce, gram, milliliter).
2. Determine the cost for the prescription quantity (e.g., 14, 30, 100).
3. Apply the markup first.
4. Apply the fees (e.g., dispensing, compounding, professional).

If a customer is eligible for discounts—senior citizen, coupons, or quantity purchase—they will always be applied after the selling price is determined. Likewise, co-pays will always be applied after the selling price is determined and discounts are applied. Co-pays are the amount of money the insurance company does not pay for. The customer is responsible for this portion and pays it when he or she picks up the prescription.

■ **EXAMPLE 8**

Joe's Pharmacy gives senior citizens a 5% discount. How much will a senior citizen pay for the prescription filled in Example 7? How much would a senior citizen pay if his or her co-pay is 10%?

$124.60 − (124.60 × 0.05) = $124.60 − $6.23 = $118.37
$118.37 × 10% = $11.84 co-pay

Practice Problems 9.2

Calculate the selling price for the following prescriptions using the information provided.

Joe's Pharmacy

Markup percent = 18%

Dispensing fee = $6

Compounding fee = $60/hr

Senior discount = 10%

1. Furosemide 40 mg #100; Cost = $95/500 tablets
2. Ranitidine 150 mg #30; Cost = $126/30 tablets
3. Digoxin 0.25 mg #90; Cost = $52/100 tablets, patient is a senior citizen
4. Camphor   10 mL $3.20
   Glycerin   20 mL $2.50
   Zinc oxide   45 g $12.00
   Vitamin A ointment 45 g $6.00
   Compounding time = 15 min
5. Promethazine syrup w/codeine 6 oz; Cost = $19.20/16 oz
6. Amoxicillin 500 mg #28; Cost = $125/500 capsules
7. Clindamycin 300 mg #42; Cost = $108/60 capsules
8. Lanolin cream   30 g $4.80
   Vitamin E oil   10 mL $6.00
   Zinc oxide   60 g $12.20
   Talc powder   30 g $15.00
   Compoundi ng time = 20 min, customer has a 5% coupon
9. Regular insulin 10 mL #3 bottles; Cost = $22/bottle, patient is a senior citizen
10. Lovastatin 20 mg #60; Cost = $216/120 tablets

INSURANCE REIMBURSEMENT

Insurance companies reimburse pharmacies for prescriptions dispensed to their clients based on the AWP pricing of medications. The AWP is the average price charged by wholesalers for a medication. Insurance companies will pay the AWP minus a percentage plus a dispensing fee. Every insurance company has a different pricing structure.

■ **EXAMPLE 9**

Insurance A pays AWP − 8% + $5.00 dispensing fee per prescription. Insurance B pays AWP − 7% + $6.00 dispensing fee. Which company will reimburse more for a prescription with an AWP of $120?

A = $120.00 − (120 × 0.08) + $5.00 = $120.00 − $9.60 + $5.00 = $115.40
B = $120.00 − (120 × 0.07) + $6.00 = $120.00 − $8.40 + $6.00 = $117.60

Some insurance companies reimburse using a system called capitation. These insurance companies pay a flat fee every month to a pharmacy no matter how many of its clients frequent that pharmacy. The fee is set by contract and is usually renegotiated annually. A pharmacy might receive $5000 monthly from Insurance A. If the pharmacy submits $4000 in claims, they will still receive $5000. On the other hand, if they submit $6000, they will receive only $5000. The goal of the pharmacy and the insurance company is to try and break even at the end of the year. Averages from previous years are used to determine the monthly fee.

Practice Problems 9.3

1. Joe's Pharmacy receives a monthly capitation fee of $5000 from Insurance Company Z. This month he processed weekly claims of $1200, $700, $1400, and $1000. How much profit/loss did Joe record?

2. Insurance A reimburses prescription claims for AWP − 7% + $4 per prescription. What is the total reimbursement for three prescriptions having a total AWP of $380?

3. Which company has a better reimbursement rate? The claim is $95.
   a. Insurance X = AWP − 4% + $2 per prescription
   b. Insurance Y = AWP − 10% + $4 per prescription

4. How much will Joe's Pharmacy receive for reimbursement on claims submitted to Insurance B that have a total AWP of $1800 for 40 prescriptions? They reimburse at AWP − 6% + $2 per prescription.

5. Joe's Pharmacy received its monthly capitation fee from Insurance Y for $3500. The claims submitted each week were $500, $700, $1200, and $1400. How much was the profit/loss for the month?

CHAPTER 9 QUIZ

1. The annual inventory for Pharmacy X is $700,000. Their average inventory is $175,000. What is their turnover rate?

2. The turnover rate for Pharmacy Y is 5. Their average inventory is $72,000. What is their annual inventory?

3. Wholesaler T gives a 15% discount to pharmacies that pay their invoices within 15 days. Joe's Pharmacy always pays their invoices in time to receive the discount. They purchased a 100-capsule bottle of indomethacin 50 mg. What is the cost of that bottle if the AWP is $185?

4. Joe's Pharmacy dispensed acetaminophen w/codeine #3, 40 tablets. The selling price was $23.40. They cost of the medication was $16.20. What is the gross profit?

5. Joe's Pharmacy dispensed azithromycin 250 mg #14 tablets for $26.40. The cost of the medication was $14.20. The dispensing costs were $9.30. What is the net profit?

   For the following prescriptions, use the information below:

   Markup = 12% for AWP less than $100

   Markup = $5 for AWP $100 or more

   Dispensing fee = $6 per prescription

   Dispensing cost = $7.50

   Compounding fee = $60 per hour

   Senior citizen discount = 10%

6. Dispense #40 alprazolam 0.5 mg tablets; AWP = $48/100 tablets

   a. What is the selling price?

   b. What is the gross profit?

   c. What is the net profit?

7. Dispense cefaclor 250 mg/5 mL 150 mL bottle; AWP = $102 per bottle

   a. What is the selling price?

   b. What is the gross profit?

   c. What is the net profit?

8. Dispense the following compounded prescription:

   Betamethasone 1%   15 g   AWP = $15.40

   Bacitracin ointment 15 g   AWP = $6.10

   Aquaphor Ointment 30 g   AWP = $4.50

   Compounding time = 10 min

   a. What is the selling price?

   b. What is the selling price for a senior citizen?

   c. What is the gross profit?

   d. What is the net profit?

9. Insurance Company A reimburses AWP − 7% + $2.50 per prescription. How much is Joe's reimbursement for:

   a. Prescription in Problem 6?

   b. Prescription in Problem 7?

   c. Prescription in Problem 8?

10. Insurance B reimburses AWP − 4% + $2 per prescription. How much is Joe's reimbursement for:

   a. Prescription in Problem 6?

   b. Prescription in Problem 7?

   c. Prescription in Problem 8?

Answer Keys

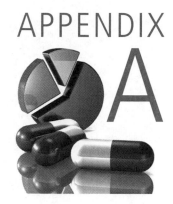

CHAPTER 1

Practice Problems 1.1

Convert the Arabic to the Roman.

1. 2010 = MMX
    1000 + 1000 + 10
      M   M   X

2. 1949 = MCMXLIX
    1000 + (1000 − 100) + (50 − 10) + (10 − 1)
      M   M   C   L   X   X   I

3. 24 = XXIV
    10 + 10 + (5 − 1)
     X   X   V   I

4. 520 = DXX
    500 + 10 + 10
      D   X   X

5. 13 = XIII
    10 + 1 + 1 + 1
     X   I   I   I

6. 93 = XCIII
    (100 − 10) + 1 + 1 + 1
      C   X   I   I   I

7. 42 = XLII
    (50 − 10) + 1 + 1
      L   X   I   I

8. 375 = CCCLXXV
    100 + 100 + 100 + 50 + 10 + 10 + 5
      C   C   C   L   X   X   V

9. 6 = VI
    5 + 1
     V I

10. 787 = DCCLXXXVII
    500 + 100 + 100 + 50 + 10 + 10 + 10 + 5 + 1 + 1
      D   C   C   L   X   X   X   V   I   I

11. 400 = CD
    500 − 100
      D   C

12. 231 = CCXXXI
    100 + 100 + 10 + 10 + 10 + 1
      C   C   X   X   X   I

13. 86 = LXXXVI
    50 + 10 + 10 + 10 + 5 + 1
      L   X   X   X   V   I

14. 66 = LXVI   50 + 10 + 5 + 1
                     L   C   V   I

15. 39 = XXXIX   10 + 10 + 10 + (10 − 1)
                     X   X   X   X   I

16. 161 = CLXI   100 + 50 + 10 + 1
                     C   L   X   I

17. 684 = DCLXXXIV   500 + 100 + 50 + 10 + 10 + 10 + (5 − 1)
                     D   C   L   X   X   X   V   I

18. 57 = LVII   50 + 5 + 1 + 1
                     L   V   I   I

19. 1496 = MCDXCVI   1000 + (500 − 100) + (100 − 10) + 5 + 1
                     M   D   C   C   X   V   I

20. 999 = CMXCIX   (1000 − 100) + (100 − 10) + (10 − 1)
                      M   C   C   X   X   I

21. 315 = CCCXV   100 + 100 + 100 + 10 + 5
                     C   C   C   X   V

22. 18 = XVIII   10 + 5 + 1 + 1 + 1
                     X   V   I   I   I

23. 540 = DXL   500 + (50 − 10)
                     D   L   X

24. 77 = LXXVII   50 + 10 + 10 + 5 + 1 + 1
                     L   X   X   V   I   I

25. 104 = CIV   100 + (5 − 1)
                     C   V   I

Convert the Roman to the Arabic.

26. MMVII = 2007   1000 + 1000 + 5 + 1 + 1
                     M   M   V   I   I

27. dxxiv = 524   500 + 10 + 10 + (5 − 1)
                     D   X   X   V   I

28. cix = 109   100 + (10 − 1)
                     C   X   I

29. LIII = 53   50 + 1 + 1 + 1
                     L   I   I   I

30. XLIX = 49   (50 − 10) + (10 − 1)
                      L   X   X   I

31. iv = 4   5 − 1
                     V   I

32. viii = 8   5 + 1 + 1 + 1
                     V   I   I   I

33. CCCXXIV = 324   100 + 100 + 100 + 10 + 10 + (5 − 1)
                     C   C   C   X   X   V   I

34. LXI = 61   50 + 10 + 1
                 L   X   I

35. dc = 600   500 + 100
                 D   C

36. MCDLVI = 1456   1000 + (500 − 100) + 50 + 5 + 1
                 M   D   C   L V I

37. vi = 6   5 + 1
                 V I

38. xxxvi = 36   10 + 10 + 10 + 5 + 1
                 X X X V I

39. iii = 3   1 + 1 + 1
                 I I I

40. LXXV = 75   50 + 10 + 10 + 5
                 L X X V

41. ccxxiv = 224   100 + 100 + 10 + 10 + (5 − 1)
                 C C X X V I

42. mmmcccxxix = 3329   1000 + 1000 + 1000 + 100 + 100 + 100 + 10 + 10 + (10 − 1)
                 M M M C C C X X X I

43. dxliv = 544   500 + (50 − 10) + (5 − 1)
                 D L X V I

44. CCL = 250   100 + 100 + 50
                 C C L

45. mv = 1005   1000 + 5
                 M V

46. XXI = 21   10 + 10 + 1
                 X X I

47. xliii = 43   (50 − 10) + 1 + 1 + 1
                 L X I I I

48. MCMLXXXII = 1982   1000 + (1000 − 100) + 50 + 10 + 10 + 10 + 1 + 1
                 M M C V X X X I I

49. xxviii = 28   10 + 10 + 5 + 1 + 1 + 1
                 X X V I I I

50. MDCCXCVI = 1796   1000 + 500 + 100 + 100 + (100 − 10) + 5 + 1
                 M D C C C X V I

Practice Problems 1.2

Convert the following.

1. **2 L**
   (1 L = 1000 mL)
   2 L × 1000 = **2000 mL**

2. **3000 mL**
   (1 mL = 1/1000 L)
   3000 mL ÷ 1000 = **3 L**

3. **1 L**
   (1 L = 1000 mL)
   1 L × 1000 = 1000 mL
   (1 mL = 1000 mcL)
   1000 mL × 1000 = **1,000,000 mcL**

4. **3 mL** = 3 mL × 1000 = **3,000 mcL**

5. **100 mcL**
   (1 mcL = 1/1000 mL)
   100 mcL ÷ 1000 = 0.1 mL
   (1 mL = 1/1000 L)
   0.1 mL ÷ 1000 = **0.0001 L**

6. **500 mL** = 500 mL ÷ 1000 = **0.5 L**

7. **500 mcL** = 500 mcL ÷ 1000 = **0.5 mL**

8. **1000 L**
   (1 L = 1 kL)
   1000 L ÷ 1000 = **1 kL**

9. **540 L**
   540 L ÷ 1000 = **0.54 kL**

10. **30 mL**
    (1 mL = 1000 mcL)
    30 mL × 1000 = **30,000 mcL**

11. **350,000 mcL**
    (1 mcL = 1/1000 mL)
    350,000 mcL ÷ 1000 = 350 mL
    (1 mL = 1/1000 L)
    350 mL ÷ 1000 = **0.35 L**

12. **1500 mL**
    (1 mL = 1000 mcL)
    1500 mL × 1000 = **1,500,000 mcL**

Practice Problems 1.3

Convert the following.

1. **2 gm**
   (1 gm = 1000 mg)
   2 gm × 1000 = 2000 mg
   (1 mg = 1000 mcg)
   2000 mg × 1000 = **2,000,000 mcg**

2. **1 mg** = 1 × 1000 = **1000 mcg**

3. **100 mg**
   (1 mg = 1/1000 g)
   100 mg ÷ 1000 = **0.1 g**

4. **2 kg** = 2 × 1000 = **2000 g**

5. **5 kg**
   (1 kg = 1000 g)
   5 kg × 1000 = 5000 g
   (1 g = 1000 mg)
   5000 g × 1000 = **5,000,000 mg**

6. **4000 mcg**
   (1 mcg = 1/1000 mg)
   4000 mcg ÷ 1000 = **4 mg**

7. **3 g**
   (1 g = 1000 mg)
   3 × 1000 = **3000 mg**

8. **500 mg**
   (1 mg = 1/1000 g)
   500 mg ÷ 1000 = **0.5 g**

9. **630 mg**
   (1 mg = 1/1000 g)
   630 mg ÷ 1000 = 0.63 g
   (1 g = 1/1000 kg)
   0.63 g ÷ 1000 = **0.00063 kg**

10. **5.4 kg**
    (1 kg = 1000 g)
    5.4 × 1000 = **5400 g**

11. **0.2 mg**
    (1 mg = 1000 mcg)
    0.2 mg × 1000 = **200 mcg**

12. **4 g**
    (1 g = 1/1000 kg)
    4 g ÷ 1000 = **0.004 kg**

13. **250 mcg**
    (1 mcg = 1/1000 mg)
    250 mcg/1000 = **0.25 mg**

14. **0.5 mg**
    (1 mg = 1000 mcg)
    0.5 mg × 1000 = **500 mcg**

15. **22 g**
    (1 g = 1000 mg)
    22 g × 1000 = **22,000 mg**

16. **320 mcg**
    (1 mcg = 1/1000 mg)
    320 ÷ 1000 = 0.32 mg
    (1 mg = 1/1000 g)
    0.32 mg ÷ 1000 = **0.00032 g**

Practice Problems 1.4

Convert the following.

1. $\frac{1}{2}$ tsp =   b. 2.5 mL

2. 3 tsp =   c. 15 mL

3. 2 pts =   a. 946 mL

4. $\frac{1}{2}$ lb =   b. 227 g
5. 3 qts =   a. 2838 mL
6. 3 tbsp =   c. 45 mL
7. 2 oz =   a. 60 mL
8. 3 oz =   b. 90 mL
9. 45 mL =   a. 1.5 oz
10. 15 mL =   b. 3 tsp
11. $\frac{1}{4}$ tsp =   c. 1.25 mL
12. 20 mL =   a. 4 tsp
13. 100 kg =   c. 220 lbs
14. 66 lbs =   b. 30 kg
15. 1892 mL =   a. $\frac{1}{2}$ gal
16. 2 qts =   b. 4 pts
17. 8 oz =   a. 48 tsp
18. 7.5 mL =   b. $1\frac{1}{2}$ tsp
19. 45 mL =   a. 3 tbsp
20. 8 oz =   c. 16 tbsp

Practice Problems 1.5

Convert the following.

1. 3 gr =   c. 195 mg
2. $\frac{1}{2}$ gr =   b. 32.5 mg
3. 4 drams =   a. $\frac{1}{2}$ oz
4. 130 mg =   a. 2 gr
5. 2 oz =   c. 60 gm
6. 30 mL =   b. 6 drams
7. 4 oz =   b. 120 g
8. $\frac{1}{2}$ dram =   b. $\frac{1}{2}$ tsp

Chapter 1 Quiz

Convert the following Arabic numerals to Roman numerals.

1. 84 = LXXXIV   50 + 10 + 10 + 10 + (5 − 1)
                        L   X   X   X   V   I

2. 310 = CCCX   100 + 100 + 100 + 10
                        C   C   C   X

3. 490 = CDXC   (500 − 100) + (100 − 10)
                                D   C   C   X

4. 19 = XIX   10 + (10 − 1)
                                X   X   I

5. 28 = XXVIII   10 + 10 + 5 + 1 + 1 + 1
                                X   X   V   I   I   I

Convert the following Roman numerals to Arabic numerals.

1. MCMXCVI = 1996   1000 + (1000 − 100) + (100 − 10) + 5 + 1
                                M   M   C   C   X   V   I

2. CCXXXIV = 234   100 + 100 + 10 + 10 + 10 + (5 − 1)
                                C   C   X   X   X   V   I

3. XCV = 95   (100 − 10) + 5
                                C   X   V

4. MMIX = 2009   1000 + 1000 + (10 − 1)
                                M   M   X   I

5. DCCC = 800   500 + 100 + 100 + 100
                                D   C   C   C

Perform the following conversions.

1. **3 L**
    (1 L = 1000 mL)
    3 L × 1000 = **3000 mL**

2. **2 g**
    (1 g = 1000 mg)
    2 g × 1000 = 2000 mg
    (1 mg = 1000 mcg)
    2000 mg × 1000 = **2,000,000 mcg**

3. **500 mL**
    (1 mL = 1/1000 L)
    500 ÷ 1000 = **0.5 L**

4. **3 kg**
    (1 kg = 1000 g)
    3 kg × 1000 = 3000 g
    (1 g = 1000 mg)
    3000 g × 1000 = **3,000,000 mg**

5. **5,000 mcL**
    (1 mcL = 1/1000 mL)
    5000 mcL ÷ 1000 = 5 mL
    (1 mL = 1/1000 L)
    5 mL ÷ 1000 = **0.005 L**

6. 700 mg
    (1 mg = 1000 mcg)
    700 mg × 1000 = **700,000 mcg**

7. **1.5 L**
   (1 L = 1000 mL)
   1.5 L × 1000 = **1500 mL**

8. **650 mcg**
   (1 mcg = 1/1000 mg)
   650 ÷ 1000 = **0.65 mg**

9. **100 mL**
   (1 mL = 1000 mcL)
   100 mL × 1000 = **100,000 mcL**

10. **3500 g**
    (1 g = 1/1000 kg)
    3500 g ÷ 1000 = **3.5 kg**

11. **2 L**
    (1 L = 1000 mL)
    2 L × 1000 = 2000 mL
    (1 mL = 1000 mcL)
    2000 mL × 1000 = **2,000,000 mcL**

12. **4.5 g**
    (1 g = 1000 mg)
    4.5 g × 1000 = **4500 mg**

13. **300 mL**
    (1 mL = 1000 mcL)
    300 mL × 1000 = **300,000 mcL**

14. **5 kg**
    (1 kg = 1000 g)
    5 kg × 1000 = **5000 g**

15. **8,000 mcL**
    (1 mcL = 1/1000 mL)
    8000 mcL ÷ 1000 = **8 mL**

16. **450 mg**
    (1 mg = 1/1000 g)
    450 mg ÷ 1000 = **0.450 g**

17. **1300 mL**
    (1 mL = 1/1000 L)
    1300 mL ÷ 1000 = **1.3 L**

18. **6 g**
    (1 g = 1000 mg)
    6 g × 1000 = 6000 mg
    (1 mg = 1000 mcg)
    6000 mg × 1000 = **6,000,000 mcg**

19. **4.2 L**
    (1 L = 1000 mL)
    4.2 L × 1000 = **4200 mL**

20. **8200 mg**
    (1 mg = 1/1000 g)
    8200 mg ÷ 1000 = **8.2 g**

Convert the following household measures.

1. **2 tsp**
   (1 tsp = 5 mL)
   2 tsp × 5 = **10 mL**

2. **2 pts**
   (1 pt = 473 mL)
   2 pts × 473 = **946 mL**

3. **2 lbs**
   (1 lb = 454 g)
   2 lbs × 454 = **908 g**

4. **2 qts**
   (1 quart = 946 mL)
   2 qts × 946 = **1892 mL**

5. **3 tbsp**
   (1 tbsp = 15 mL)
   3 tbsp × 15 = **45 mL**

6. **176 lbs =**
   (1 kg = 2.2 lbs)
   176 lbs ÷ 2.2 = **80 kg**

7. **6 oz**
   (1 oz = 30 mL)
   6 oz × 30 = 180 mL
   (1 tsp = 5 mL)
   180 mL ÷ 5 = **36 tsp**

8. **5 gr**
   (1 gr = 65 mg)
   5 gr × 65 = **325 mg**

9. **5 oz**
   (1 oz = 30 g)
   5 oz × 30 = **150 g**

10. **650 mg**
    (1 mg = 1/65 gr)
    650 mg ÷ 65 = **10 gr**

11. **8 oz**
    (1 oz = 30 mL)
    8 oz × 30 = **240 mL**

12. **25 kg**
    (1 kg = 2.2 lbs)
    25 kg × 2.2 = **55 lbs**

13. **15 mL**
    (1 mL = 1/5 tsp)
    15 mL ÷ 5 = **3 tsp**

14. **60 mL**
    (1 mL = 1/15 tbsp)
    60 mL ÷ 15 = **4 tbsp**

15. **120 mL**
    (1 mL = 1/30 mL)
    120 mL ÷ 30 = **4 oz**

16. **180 g**
    (1 g = 1/30 oz)
    180 g ÷ 30 = **6 oz**

17. **7.5 mL**
    (1 mL = 1/5 tsp)
    7.5 mL ÷ 5 = **$1\frac{1}{2}$ tsp**

18. **$\frac{1}{4}$ tsp**
    (1 tsp = 5 mL)
    $\frac{1}{4}$ tsp × 5 = **1.25 mL**

19. **45 mL**
    (1 mL = 1/15 tbsp)
    45 mL ÷ 15 = **3 tbsp**

20. **275 lbs**
    (1 lb = 2.2 kg)
    275 lbs ÷ 2.2 = **125 kg**

CHAPTER 2

Practice Problems 2.1

Simplify the answer to a proper fraction in its simplest terms.

1. $\dfrac{4}{5} + \dfrac{4}{5} = \dfrac{4+4}{5} = \dfrac{8}{5} = 1\dfrac{3}{5}$

2. $\dfrac{3}{8} + \dfrac{2}{8} = \dfrac{3+2}{8} = \dfrac{5}{8}$

3. $\dfrac{5}{12} + \dfrac{6}{24} = \left(\dfrac{5}{12} \times \dfrac{2}{2}\right) + \dfrac{6}{24} = \dfrac{10}{24} + \dfrac{6}{24} = \dfrac{16}{24} \div \dfrac{8}{8} = \dfrac{2}{3}$

4. $\dfrac{1}{3} + \dfrac{4}{9} = \left(\dfrac{1}{3} \times \dfrac{3}{3}\right) + \dfrac{4}{9} = \dfrac{3}{9} + \dfrac{4}{9} = \dfrac{7}{9}$

5. $\dfrac{8}{27} + \dfrac{7}{8} = \left(\dfrac{8}{27} \times \dfrac{8}{8}\right) + \left(\dfrac{7}{8} \times \dfrac{27}{27}\right) = \dfrac{64}{216} + \dfrac{189}{216} = \dfrac{253}{216} = 1\dfrac{37}{216}$

6. $\dfrac{9}{7} + \dfrac{2}{7} = \dfrac{11}{7} = 1\dfrac{4}{7}$

7. $\dfrac{6}{7} - \dfrac{2}{7} = \dfrac{4}{7}$

8. $\dfrac{7}{9} - \dfrac{1}{3} = \dfrac{7}{9} - \left(\dfrac{1}{3} \times \dfrac{3}{3}\right) = \dfrac{7}{9} - \dfrac{3}{9} = \dfrac{4}{9}$

9. $\dfrac{7}{15} + \dfrac{4}{60} = \left(\dfrac{7}{15} \times \dfrac{4}{4}\right) + \dfrac{4}{60} = \dfrac{28}{60} + \dfrac{4}{60} = \dfrac{32}{60} \div \dfrac{4}{4} = \dfrac{8}{15}$

10. $\dfrac{3}{13} + \dfrac{4}{7} = \left(\dfrac{3}{13} \times \dfrac{7}{7}\right) + \left(\dfrac{4}{7} \times \dfrac{13}{13}\right) = \dfrac{21}{91} + \dfrac{52}{91} = \dfrac{73}{91}$

11. $4\dfrac{3}{4} + \dfrac{7}{4} = \left(\dfrac{4 \times 4 + 3}{4}\right) + \dfrac{7}{4} = \dfrac{19}{4} + \dfrac{7}{4} = \dfrac{26}{4} = 6\dfrac{2}{4} = 6\dfrac{1}{2}$

12. $\dfrac{8}{5} + 2\dfrac{1}{10} = \left(\dfrac{8}{5} \times \dfrac{2}{2}\right) + \left(\dfrac{2 \times 10 + 1}{10}\right) = \dfrac{16}{10} + \dfrac{21}{10} = \dfrac{37}{10} = 3\dfrac{7}{10}$

13. $5\dfrac{2}{3} - 2\dfrac{1}{3} = \left(\dfrac{3 \times 5 + 2}{3}\right) - \left(\dfrac{3 \times 2 + 1}{3}\right) = \dfrac{17}{3} - \dfrac{7}{3} = \dfrac{10}{3} = 3\dfrac{1}{3}$

14. $\dfrac{12}{7} + \dfrac{3}{7} = \dfrac{15}{7} = 2\dfrac{1}{7}$

15. $\dfrac{6}{21} + \dfrac{4}{21} = \dfrac{10}{21}$

Practice Problems 2.2

Solve the following equations and simplify.

1. $\dfrac{5}{7} \times \dfrac{4}{8} = \dfrac{5 \times 4}{7 \times 8} = \dfrac{20}{56} \div \dfrac{4}{4} = \dfrac{5}{14}$

2. $\dfrac{2}{4} \times \dfrac{8}{13} = \dfrac{2 \times 8}{4 \times 13} = \dfrac{16}{52} \div \dfrac{4}{4} = \dfrac{4}{13}$

3. $\dfrac{12}{13} \times \dfrac{3}{5} = \dfrac{12 \times 3}{13 \times 5} = \dfrac{36}{65}$

4. $\dfrac{3}{7} \times \dfrac{2}{9} \times \dfrac{1}{4} = \dfrac{3 \times 2 \times 1}{7 \times 9 \times 4} = \dfrac{6}{252} = \dfrac{1}{42}$

5. $\dfrac{1}{4} \times \dfrac{2}{3} \times \dfrac{5}{6} = \dfrac{1 \times 2 \times 5}{4 \times 3 \times 6} = \dfrac{10}{72} = \dfrac{5}{36}$

6. $2\dfrac{3}{4} \times \dfrac{7}{8} \times 1\dfrac{1}{4} = \left(\dfrac{4 \times 2 + 3}{4}\right) \times \dfrac{7}{8} \times \left(\dfrac{4 \times 1 + 1}{4}\right) = \dfrac{11 \times 7 \times 5}{4 \times 8 \times 4} = \dfrac{385}{128} = 3\dfrac{1}{128}$

7. $\dfrac{11}{12} \div \dfrac{3}{4} = \dfrac{11}{12} \times \dfrac{4}{3} = \dfrac{11 \times 4}{12 \times 3} = \dfrac{44}{36} = 1\dfrac{8}{36} = 1\dfrac{2}{9}$

8. $\dfrac{5}{6} \div \dfrac{1}{3} = \dfrac{5}{6} \times \dfrac{3}{1} = \dfrac{5 \times 3}{6 \times 1} = \dfrac{15}{6} = 2\dfrac{3}{6} = 2\dfrac{1}{2}$

9. $9 \div \dfrac{4}{5} = \dfrac{9}{1} \times \dfrac{5}{4} = \dfrac{9 \times 5}{1 \times 4} = \dfrac{45}{4} = 11\dfrac{1}{4}$

10. $\dfrac{1}{5} \div 6 = \dfrac{1}{5} \times \dfrac{1}{6} = \dfrac{1}{30}$

11. $3\dfrac{1}{2} \div \dfrac{7}{8} = \left(\dfrac{2 \times 3 + 1}{2}\right) \times \dfrac{8}{7} = \dfrac{7 \times 8}{2 \times 7} = \dfrac{56}{14} = 4$

12. $2\dfrac{3}{4} \div 1\dfrac{5}{8} = \left(\dfrac{4 \times 2 + 3}{4}\right) \times \left(\dfrac{8}{8 \times 1 + 5}\right) = \dfrac{11 \times 8}{4 \times 13} = \dfrac{88}{52} = 1\dfrac{36}{52} = 1\dfrac{9}{13}$

Practice Problems 2.3

Round to the correct decimal position.

1. $23.4 \times 42.87 = 1003.158 = 1003.2$

2. $8.56 \times 39.2 = 335.552 = 335.6$

3. $146 \times 15.58 = 2274.68 = 2275$

4. $1.4756 \times 2.4 = 3.5414 = 3.5$

5. $3.4 \times 4.21 \times 1.8 = 25.7652 = 25.8$

6. $4.56 \div 2.3 = 456 \div 230 = 1.9826 = 2.0$

7. $45.98 \div 9.135 = 45980 \div 9135 = 5.0334 = 5.03$

8. $\dfrac{7.34}{4.9} = 734 \div 490 = 1.4980 = 1.5$

9. $\dfrac{5.3214}{3.87} = 53214 \div 38700 = 1.375 = 1.38$

10. $24 \div 4.34 = 2400 \div 434 = 5.53 = 6$

Practice Problems 2.4

Determine the significant figures—final zeros are *not* significant.

1. $0.254 = 3$
2. $1.085 = 4$
3. $43.2 = 3$
4. $2.0001 = 5$
5. $3.0 = 1$
6. $902 = 3$

7. $5439.1 = 5$
8. $1.2040 = 4$
9. $22{,}432.2 = 6$
10. $0.0003 = 1$
11. $700 = 1$
12. $0.019040 = 4$

Round to three significant figures.

13. $57.82 = 57.8$
14. $49.074 = 49.1$
15. $0.5486 = 0.549$

16. $0.00486 = 0.00486$
17. $1.438 = 1.44$
18. $1.899 = 1.90$

Chapter 2 Quiz

Perform the following calculations. Simplify when possible.

1. $\dfrac{2}{4} + \dfrac{2}{3} = \left(\dfrac{2}{4} \times \dfrac{3}{3}\right) + \left(\dfrac{2}{3} \times \dfrac{4}{4}\right) = \dfrac{6}{12} + \dfrac{8}{12} = \dfrac{14}{12} = 1\dfrac{2}{12} = 1\dfrac{1}{6}$

2. $\dfrac{4}{5} + \dfrac{7}{8} = \left(\dfrac{4}{5} \times \dfrac{8}{8}\right) + \left(\dfrac{7}{8} \times \dfrac{5}{5}\right) = \dfrac{32}{40} + \dfrac{35}{40} = \dfrac{67}{40} = 1\dfrac{27}{40}$

3. $\dfrac{6}{20} + \dfrac{4}{10} + \dfrac{4}{5} = \dfrac{6}{20} + \left(\dfrac{4}{10} \times \dfrac{2}{2}\right) + \left(\dfrac{4}{5} \times \dfrac{4}{4}\right) = \dfrac{6}{20} + \dfrac{8}{20} + \dfrac{16}{20} = \dfrac{30}{20} = 1\dfrac{10}{20} = 1\dfrac{1}{2}$

4. $\dfrac{9}{14} - \dfrac{3}{14} = \dfrac{9-3}{14} = \dfrac{6}{14} = \dfrac{3}{7}$

5. $2\dfrac{5}{6} + 3\dfrac{1}{4} = \left(\dfrac{2 \times 6 + 5}{6}\right) + \left(\dfrac{3 \times 4 + 1}{4}\right) = \dfrac{17}{6} + \dfrac{13}{4} = \left(\dfrac{17}{6} \times \dfrac{2}{2}\right) + \left(\dfrac{13}{4} \times \dfrac{3}{3}\right) =$

   $\dfrac{34}{12} + \dfrac{39}{12} = \dfrac{73}{12} = 6\dfrac{1}{12}$

6. $\dfrac{5}{6} \times \dfrac{3}{8} = \dfrac{5 \times 3}{6 \times 8} = \dfrac{15}{48} \div \dfrac{3}{3} = \dfrac{5}{16}$

7. $\dfrac{10}{75} \times \dfrac{20}{100} = \dfrac{10 \times 20}{75 \times 100} = \dfrac{200}{7500} \div \dfrac{100}{100} = \dfrac{2}{75}$

8. $\dfrac{7}{15} \times \dfrac{3}{4} = \dfrac{7 \times 3}{15 \times 4} = \dfrac{21}{60} \div \dfrac{3}{3} = \dfrac{7}{20}$

9. $8 \div \dfrac{2}{3} = \dfrac{8}{1} \times \dfrac{3}{2} = \dfrac{8 \times 3}{1 \times 2} = \dfrac{24}{2} = 12$

10. $3\dfrac{1}{3} \times 4\dfrac{1}{4} = \dfrac{3 \times 3 + 1}{3} \times \dfrac{4 \times 4 + 1}{4} = \dfrac{10 \times 17}{3 \times 4} = \dfrac{170}{12} = 14\dfrac{2}{12} = 14\dfrac{1}{6}$

11. $\dfrac{5}{9} + \dfrac{2}{9} = \dfrac{5 + 2}{9} = \dfrac{7}{9}$

12. $\dfrac{2}{15} + \dfrac{8}{15} = \dfrac{2 + 8}{15} = \dfrac{10}{15} \div \dfrac{5}{5} = \dfrac{2}{3}$

13. $\dfrac{7}{8} - \dfrac{3}{4} = \dfrac{7}{8} - \left(\dfrac{3}{4} \times \dfrac{2}{2}\right) = \dfrac{7}{8} - \dfrac{6}{8} = \dfrac{1}{8}$

14. $\dfrac{5}{8} - \dfrac{1}{3} = \left(\dfrac{5}{8} \times \dfrac{3}{3}\right) - \left(\dfrac{1}{3} \times \dfrac{8}{8}\right) = \dfrac{15}{24} - \dfrac{8}{24} = \dfrac{7}{24}$

15. $4\dfrac{2}{13} + 3\dfrac{7}{26} = \left(\dfrac{(4 \times 13 + 2)}{13} \times \dfrac{2}{2}\right) + \dfrac{3 \times 26 + 7}{26} = \dfrac{108}{26} + \dfrac{85}{26} = \dfrac{193}{26} = 7\dfrac{11}{26}$

16. $\dfrac{11}{14} \times \dfrac{1}{4} = \dfrac{11 \times 1}{14 \times 4} = \dfrac{11}{56}$

17. $\dfrac{2}{3} \times \dfrac{1}{4} \times \dfrac{7}{8} = \dfrac{2 \times 1 \times 7}{3 \times 4 \times 8} = \dfrac{14}{96} \div \dfrac{2}{2} = \dfrac{7}{48}$

18. $\dfrac{5}{8} \div \dfrac{1}{2} = \dfrac{5}{8} \times \dfrac{2}{1} = \dfrac{10}{8} = 1\dfrac{2}{8} = 1\dfrac{1}{4}$

19. $\dfrac{2}{7} \div 4 = \dfrac{2}{7} \times \dfrac{1}{4} = \dfrac{2}{28} = \dfrac{1}{14}$

20. $6\dfrac{1}{4} \div 3\dfrac{1}{3} = \dfrac{4 \times 6 + 1}{4} \div \dfrac{3 \times 3 + 1}{3} = \dfrac{25}{4} \times \dfrac{3}{10} = \dfrac{75}{40} = 1\dfrac{35}{40} = 1\dfrac{7}{8}$

Perform the following calculations. Round to the proper decimal position.

1. $23.6 + 42.87 = 66.47 = 66.5$
2. $346.42 + 2.68 + 49.572 = 398.672 = 398.67$
3. $423.73 - 284.6 = 139.13 = 139.1$
4. $26.84 - 14.82 = 12.02$
5. $3.1 \times 6.82 = 21.142 = 21.1$
6. $7.42 \div 3.6 = 2.0611 = 2.1$
7. $9.8624 \div 4.36 = 2.262 = 2.26$
8. $17 \div 2.46 = 6.9106 = 7$
9. $5.62 \times 3.9 = 21.918 = 21.9$
10. $8.92 \times 2.6 = 23.192 = 23.2$

Determine the significant figures—final zeros are *not* significant.

1. $0.426 = 3$
2. $3.028 = 4$
3. $7326.4 = 5$
4. $1.8604 = 5$
5. $7.0 = 1$

Round to three significant figures.

1. $52.083 = 52.1$
2. $1.377 = 1.38$
3. $0.6491 = 0.649$
4. $1.888 = 1.89$
5. $234.2 = 234$

CHAPTER 3

Practice Problems 3.1

Convert the following ratios to fractions and simplify to the lowest term possible.

1. $3{:}9 = \dfrac{3}{9} = \dfrac{1}{3}$

2. $2{:}5 = \dfrac{2}{5}$

3. $5{:}20 = \dfrac{5}{20} = \dfrac{1}{4}$

4. $1{:}10 = \dfrac{1}{10}$

5. $6{:}7 = \dfrac{6}{7}$

6. $14{:}23 = \dfrac{14}{23}$

7. $3{:}4 = \dfrac{3}{4}$

8. $8{:}3 = \dfrac{8}{3}$

9. $1{:}18 = \dfrac{1}{18}$

10. $4{:}25 = \dfrac{4}{25}$

Convert the following fractions to ratios and simplify to the lowest term possible.

11. $\dfrac{3}{4} = 3{:}4$

12. $\dfrac{4}{6} = 4{:}6 = 2{:}3$

13. $\dfrac{1}{8} = 1{:}8$

14. $\dfrac{2}{1000} = 2{:}1000 = 1{:}500$

15. $\dfrac{15}{30} = 15{:}30 = 1{:}2$

16. $\dfrac{1}{10,000} = 1{:}10,000$

17. $\dfrac{3}{9} = 3{:}9 = 1{:}3$

18. $\dfrac{10}{12} = 10{:}12 = 5{:}6$

19. $\dfrac{5}{9} = 5{:}9$

20. $\dfrac{7}{49} = 7{:}49 = 1{:}7$

Determine the ratio for the following drugs and simplify to the lowest term possible.

21. 750 mg tablet of clarithromycin = 1:750

22. 10 mg capsule dicyclomine = 1:10

23. 125 mg of amoxicillin in 5 mL = 125:5 = 25:1

24. 300 mg of ranitidine in 2 mL = 300:2 = 150:1

25. 20 mg of diphenhydramine in 1 g = 20:1000 = 1:50

Write a ratio equation for the following problems.

26. Dispense cimetidine 400 mg per dose; on hand is 200 mg tablets

$$\dfrac{400 \text{ mg}}{1} = \dfrac{200 \text{ mg}}{x}$$

27. Dispense 10 mg metoclopramide per dose; on hand is 5 mg/mL

$$\dfrac{10 \text{ mg}}{x} = \dfrac{5 \text{ mg}}{1 \text{ mL}}$$

28. Dispense 250 mg dicloxacillin per dose; on hand is 500 mg/5 mL

$$\frac{250 \text{ mg}}{x} = \frac{500 \text{ mg}}{5 \text{ mL}}$$

Define the following ratios.

29. 1:2000 w/w = 1 g per 2000 g
30. 2:500 w/v = 2 g per 500 mL

Practice Problems 3.2

Solve for x.

1. $\frac{4}{12} = \frac{x}{3}$
   $x = (4 \times 3) \div 12 = 1$

2. $\frac{x}{42} = \frac{1}{7}$
   $x = (42 \times 1) \div 7 = 6$

3. $\frac{0.5}{4} = \frac{x}{16}$
   $x = (0.5 \times 6) \div 4 = 0.75$

4. $\frac{250}{5} = \frac{375}{x}$
   $x = (5 \times 375) \div 250 = 7.5$

5. $\frac{7}{10} = \frac{x}{9}$
   $x = (7 \times 9) \div 10 = 6.3$

6. $\frac{21}{x} = \frac{105}{5}$
   $x = (21 \times 5) \div 105 = 1$

7. $\frac{330}{5} = \frac{495}{x}$
   $x = (5 \times 495) \div 330 = 7.5$

8. $\frac{x}{50} = \frac{20}{250}$
   $x = (50 \times 20) \div 250 = 4$

9. $\frac{0.5}{1} = \frac{6}{x}$
   $x = (1 \times 6) \div 0.5 = 12$

10. $\frac{375}{12} = \frac{x}{16}$
    $x = (375 \times 16) \div 12 = 500$

Convert the following weights using the proportion rule.

11. 450 mg = x g
    $$\frac{1 \text{ g}}{1000 \text{ mg}} = \frac{x}{450 \text{ mg}}$$
    $x = (1 \text{ g} \times 450 \text{ mg}) \div 1000 \text{ mg} = 0.45 \text{ g}$

12. 0.95 gm = x mg
    $$\frac{1 \text{ g}}{1000 \text{ mg}} = \frac{0.95 \text{ g}}{x}$$
    $x = (0.95 \text{ g} \times 1000 \text{ mg}) \div 1 \text{ g} = 950 \text{ mg}$

13. 2450 mg = x g
    $$\frac{1 \text{ g}}{1000 \text{ mg}} = \frac{x}{2450 \text{ mg}}$$
    $x = (1 \text{ g} \times 2450 \text{ mg}) \div 1000 \text{ mg} = 2.45 \text{ g}$

14. 2.75 mg = x mcg

$$\frac{1 \text{ mg}}{1000 \text{ mcg}} = \frac{2.75 \text{ mg}}{x}$$

$x = (1000 \text{ mcg} \times 2.75 \text{ mg}) \div 1 \text{ mg} = 2750 \text{ mcg}$

15. 540 mcg = x mg

$$\frac{1 \text{ mg}}{1000 \text{ mcg}} = \frac{x}{540 \text{ mcg}}$$

$x = (540 \text{ mcg} \times 1 \text{ mg}) \div 1000 \text{ mcg} = 0.54 \text{ mg}$

16. 65 lbs = x kg

$$\frac{1 \text{ kg}}{2.2 \text{ lbs}} = \frac{x}{65 \text{ lbs}}$$

$x = (65 \text{ lbs} \times 1 \text{ kg}) \div 2.2 \text{ lbs} = 29.5 \text{ kg}$

17. 240 kg = x lbs

$$\frac{1 \text{ kg}}{2.2 \text{ lbs}} = \frac{240 \text{ kg}}{x}$$

$x = (240 \text{ kg} \times 2.2 \text{ lbs}) \div 1 \text{ kg} = 528 \text{ lbs}$

18. 120 kg = x lbs

$$\frac{1 \text{ kg}}{2.2 \text{ lbs}} = \frac{120 \text{ kg}}{x}$$

$x = (120 \text{ kg} \times 2.2 \text{ lbs}) \div 1 \text{ kg} = 264 \text{ lbs}$

19. 132 lbs = x kg

$$\frac{1 \text{ kg}}{2.2 \text{ lbs}} = \frac{x}{132 \text{ lbs}}$$

$x = (132 \text{ lbs} \times 1 \text{ kg}) \div 2.2 = 60 \text{ kg}$

20. 22 lbs = x kg

$$\frac{1 \text{ kg}}{2.2 \text{ lbs}} = \frac{x}{22 \text{ lbs}}$$

$x = (22 \text{ lbs} \times 1 \text{ kg}) \div 2.2 \text{ lbs} = 10 \text{ kg}$

Use the proportion rule to solve for needed dosage in the following problems.

21. A prescription calls for 225 mg dose of amoxicillin every 6 hr for 10 days. The pharmacy carries 125 mg/5 mL concentration.

   a. How much is needed for each dose?

   $$\frac{125 \text{ mg}}{5 \text{ mL}} = \frac{225 \text{ mg}}{x}$$

   $x = (225 \text{ mg} \times 5 \text{ mL}) \div 125 \text{ mg} = 9 \text{ mL}$

   b. How much is needed to fill the entire prescription?

   9 mL × 4 doses (every 6 hr) = 36 mL × 10 days = 360 mL

22. Heparin comes in 5000 units/mL concentration; the patient needs a dose of 2000 units. How many mLs are needed?

$$\frac{5000 \text{ units}}{1 \text{ mL}} = \frac{2000 \text{ units}}{x}$$

$x = (2000 \text{ units} \times 1 \text{ mL}) \div 5000 \text{ units} = 0.4 \text{ mL}$

23. A patient needs 550 mg of amikacin. The pharmacy carries 500 mg/2 mL vials. How much is needed for this dose?

$$\frac{500 \text{ mg}}{2 \text{ mL}} = \frac{550 \text{ mg}}{x}$$

$x = (550 \text{ mg} \times 2 \text{ mL}) \div 500 \text{ mg} = 2.2 \text{ mL}$

24. An IV solution needs 35 mEq of potassium added. The pharmacy carries 50 mL vials with a concentration of 2 mEq/mL. How much is needed for this dose?

$$\frac{2 \text{ mEq}}{1 \text{ mL}} = \frac{35 \text{ mEq}}{x}$$

$x = (35 \text{ mEq} \times 1 \text{ mL}) \div 2 \text{ mEq} = 17.5 \text{ mL}$

25. A prescription calls for 500 mg of erythromycin. The pharmacy only carries 250 mg tablets. How many will be dispensed for each dose?

$$\frac{250 \text{ mg}}{1 \text{ tab}} = \frac{500 \text{ mg}}{x}$$

$x = (500 \text{ mg} \times 1 \text{ tab}) \div 250 \text{ mg} = 2 \text{ tabs}$

26. A physician orders furosemide 50 mg IV now for a patient. The pharmacy carries 20 mg/2 mL concentration. How much will you dispense for this dose?

$$\frac{20 \text{ mg}}{2 \text{ mL}} = \frac{50 \text{ mg}}{x}$$

$x = (50 \text{ mg} \times 2 \text{ mL}) \div 20 \text{ mg} = 5 \text{ mL}$

27. You receive a prescription for albuterol 4 mg twice a day for 14 days. The pharmacy carries 2 mg/5 mL concentration in pint bottles.

    a. How much will the patient take per dose?

    $$\frac{2 \text{ mg}}{5 \text{ mL}} = \frac{4 \text{ mg}}{x}$$

    $x = (4 \text{ mg} \times 5 \text{ mL}) \div 2 \text{ mg} = 10 \text{ mL}$

    b. How much will you dispense to fill the entire prescription?

    10 mL × 2 doses = 20 mL daily × 14 days = 280 mL

28. Propranolol 40 mg tablets are ordered for a patient. The pharmacy is out of 40 mg tablets and has only 80 mg tablets available. How many tablets will be dispensed for a 40 mg dose?

$$\frac{80\ mg}{1\ tab} = \frac{40\ mg}{x}$$

$x = (40\ mg \times 1\ tab) \div 80\ mg = \frac{1}{2}\ tab$

29. An infant needs 10 mg/kg of an antibiotic. The infant weighs 11 lbs. The antibiotic is available in 100 mg/10 mL concentration.

    a. How much does the infant weigh in kg?

    11 lbs ÷ 2.2 kg = 5 kg

    b. What is the dose needed for the infant?

    5 kg × 10 mg = 50 mg

    c. How many mLs of the antibiotic are needed for this dose?

$$\frac{100\ mg}{10\ mL} = \frac{50\ mg}{x}$$

    $x = (50\ mg \times 10\ mL) \div 100\ mg = 5\ mL$

30. A patient has a prescription for clindamycin 300 mg four times a day for 14 days. The pharmacy only carries the 150 mg capsules.

    a. How many capsules are needed per dose?

$$\frac{150\ mg}{1\ capsule} = \frac{300\ mg}{x}$$

    $x = (300\ mg \times 1\ cap) \div 150\ mg = 2\ capsules$

    b. How many capsules are needed daily?

    2 capsules × 4 doses = 8 capsules daily

    c. How many capsules are needed for the entire prescription?

    8 capsules × 14 days = 112 capsules

Practice Problems 3.3

Convert the following ratios to percents.

1. $2{:}300 = \dfrac{2}{300} = 0.00666 \times 100 = 0.67\%$

2. $3{:}4 = \dfrac{3}{4} = 0.75 \times 100 = 75\%$

3. $1{:}1000 = \dfrac{1}{1000} = 0.001 \times 100 = 0.1\%$

4. $1{:}5 = \dfrac{1}{5} = 0.2 \times 100 = 20\%$

5. $6{:}10 = \dfrac{6}{10} = 0.6 \times 100 = 60\%$

Convert the following percents to ratios and simplify to the lowest form.

6. $3\% = \dfrac{3}{100} = 3{:}100$

7. $42\% = \dfrac{42}{100} \div \dfrac{2}{2} = \dfrac{21}{50} = 21{:}50$

8. $0.5\% = \dfrac{0.5}{100} \div \dfrac{0.5}{0.5} = \dfrac{1}{200} = 1{:}200$

9. $1.6\% = \dfrac{1.6}{100} \div \dfrac{4}{4} = \dfrac{0.4}{25} = 0.4{:}25$

10. $150\% = \dfrac{150}{100} \div \dfrac{50}{50} = \dfrac{3}{2} = 3{:}2$

Convert the following fractions to percents.

11. $\dfrac{5}{7} = 5 \div 7 = 0.714 \times 100 = 71.4\%$

12. $\dfrac{2}{8} = 2 \div 8 = 0.25 \times 100 = 25\%$

13. $\dfrac{14}{52} = 14 \div 52 = 0.269 \times 100 = 26.9\%$

14. $\dfrac{0.4}{2} = 0.4 \div 2 = 0.2 \times 100 = 20\%$

15. $\dfrac{3}{4} = 3 \div 4 = 0.75 \times 100 = 75\%$

Convert the following percents to fractions and simplify to the lowest form.

16. $24\% = \dfrac{24}{100} \div \dfrac{4}{4} = \dfrac{6}{25}$

17. $0.25\% = \dfrac{0.25}{100} \div \dfrac{0.25}{0.25} = \dfrac{1}{400}$

18. $140\% = \dfrac{140}{100} \div \dfrac{20}{20} = \dfrac{7}{5} = 1\tfrac{2}{5}$

19. $1.65\% = \dfrac{1.65}{100} \div \dfrac{5}{5} = \dfrac{0.33}{20}$

20. $2\% = \dfrac{2}{100} \div \dfrac{2}{2} = \dfrac{1}{50}$

Calculate the following percents.

21. $5\% \text{ of } 50 = \dfrac{5}{100} = \dfrac{x}{50}$

$x = (5 \times 50) \div 100 = 2.5$

22. $20\% \text{ of } 60 = \dfrac{20}{100} = \dfrac{x}{60}$

$x = (20 \times 60) \div 100 = 12$

23. 18% of $42 = \dfrac{18}{100} = \dfrac{x}{42}$

$x = (18 \times 42) \div 100 = 7.56$

24. 110% of $75 = \dfrac{110}{100} = \dfrac{x}{75}$

$x = (110 \times 75) \div 100 = 82.5$

25. 0.5% of $80 = \dfrac{0.5}{100} = \dfrac{x}{80}$

$x = (0.5 \times 80) \div 100 = 0.4$

Chapter 3 Quiz

Convert the following ratios to fractions and simplify when possible.

1. $4{:}10 = \dfrac{4}{10} \div \dfrac{2}{2} = \dfrac{2}{5}$

2. $3{:}15 = \dfrac{3}{15} \div \dfrac{3}{3} = \dfrac{1}{5}$

3. $6{:}50 = \dfrac{6}{50} \div \dfrac{2}{2} = \dfrac{3}{25}$

4. $40{:}1000 = \dfrac{40}{1000} \div \dfrac{40}{40} = \dfrac{1}{25}$

5. $2{:}7 = \dfrac{2}{7}$

Convert the following fractions to ratios and simplify when possible.

1. $\dfrac{120}{700} \div \dfrac{20}{20} = \dfrac{6}{35} = 6{:}35$

2. $\dfrac{1}{9} = 1{:}9$

3. $\dfrac{5}{40} \div \dfrac{5}{5} = \dfrac{1}{8} = 1{:}8$

4. $\dfrac{1}{1000} = 1{:}1000$

5. $\dfrac{6}{240} \div \dfrac{6}{6} = \dfrac{1}{40} = 1{:}40$

Convert the following percents to ratios and simplify when possible.

1. $20\% = \dfrac{20}{100} \div \dfrac{20}{20} = \dfrac{1}{5} = 1{:}5$

2. $4\% = \dfrac{4}{100} \div \dfrac{4}{4} = \dfrac{1}{25} = 1{:}25$

3. $58\% = \dfrac{58}{100} \div \dfrac{2}{2} = \dfrac{29}{50} = 29{:}50$

4. $0.4\% = \dfrac{0.4}{100} \div \dfrac{0.4}{0.4} = \dfrac{1}{250} = 1{:}250$

5. $1.5\% = \dfrac{1.5}{100} \div \dfrac{0.5}{0.5} = \dfrac{3}{200} = 3{:}200$

Convert the following ratios to percents.

1. $2{:}3 = \dfrac{2}{3} = 0.666 \times 100 = 66.6\%$

2. $1{:}500 = \dfrac{1}{500} = 0.002 \times 100 = 0.2\%$

3. $4{:}10 = \dfrac{4}{10} \div \dfrac{2}{2} = \dfrac{2}{5} = 0.4 \times 100 = 40\%$

4. $15{:}40 = \dfrac{15}{40} \div \dfrac{5}{5} = \dfrac{3}{8} = 0.375 \times 100 = 37.5\%$

5. $1{:}1000 = \dfrac{1}{1000} = 0.001 \times 100 = 0.1\%$

Convert the following fractions to percents.

1. $\dfrac{5}{7} = 5 \div 7 = 0.714 \times 100 = 71.4\%$

2. $\dfrac{42}{100} = 42 \div 100 = 0.42 \times 100 = 42\%$

3. $\dfrac{3}{10} = 3 \div 10 = 0.3 \times 100 = 30\%$

4. $\dfrac{9}{20} = 9 \div 20 = 0.45 \times 100 = 45\%$

5. $\dfrac{0.8}{10} = 0.8 \div 10 = 0.08 \times 100 = 8\%$

Convert the following percents to fractions and simplify when possible.

1. $52\% = \dfrac{52}{100} \div \dfrac{4}{4} = \dfrac{13}{25}$

2. $3\% = \dfrac{3}{100}$

3. $110\% = \dfrac{110}{100} = \dfrac{10}{10} = \dfrac{11}{10} = 1\dfrac{1}{10}$

4. $0.4\% = \dfrac{0.4}{100} \div \dfrac{0.4}{0.4} = \dfrac{1}{250}$

5. $3.7\% = \dfrac{3.7}{100}$

Solve the following proportions.

1. $\dfrac{9}{42} = \dfrac{x}{126}$

   $x = (9 \times 126) \div 42 = 27$

2. $\dfrac{14}{x} = \dfrac{70}{85}$

   $x = (14 \times 85) \div 70 = 17$

3. $\dfrac{3}{5} = \dfrac{24}{x}$

   $x = (5 \times 24) \div 3 = 40$

4. $\dfrac{82}{x} = \dfrac{41}{68}$

   $x = (82 \times 68) \div 41 = 136$

5. $\dfrac{x}{110} = \dfrac{80}{440}$

   $x = (110 \times 80) \div 440 = 20$

6. $\dfrac{125}{5} = \dfrac{400}{x}$

   $x = (5 \times 400) \div 125 = 16$

7. $\dfrac{1500}{50} = \dfrac{x}{10}$

   $x = (1500 \times 10) \div 50 = 300$

8. $\dfrac{400}{5} = \dfrac{x}{20}$

   $x = (400 \times 20) \div 5 = 1600$

9. $\dfrac{40}{2} = \dfrac{180}{x}$

   $x = (180 \times 2) \div 40 = 9$

10. $\dfrac{1000}{10} = \dfrac{300}{x}$

    $x = (300 \times 10) \div 1000 = 3$

Solve the following problems.

1. Diazepam comes in 5 mg/mL concentration. The dose is 3 mg. How many mLs are needed for the dose?

   $\dfrac{5 \text{ mg}}{1 \text{ mL}} = \dfrac{3 \text{ mg}}{x}$

   $x = (3 \text{ mg} \times 1 \text{ mL}) \div 5 \text{ mg} = 0.6 \text{ mL}$

2. The patient needs 450 mg of clindamycin. The pharmacy stocks 300 mg/2 mL concentration. How many mLs are needed for the dose?

   $\dfrac{300 \text{ mg}}{2 \text{ mL}} = \dfrac{450 \text{ mg}}{x}$

   $x = (450 \text{ mg} \times 2 \text{ mL}) \div 300 \text{ mg} = 3 \text{ mL}$

3. An antibiotic suspension is available in 500 mg/5 mL concentration. The dose is 150 mg four times a day.

   a. How many mLs are needed for one dose?

   $\dfrac{500 \text{ mg}}{5 \text{ mL}} = \dfrac{150 \text{ mg}}{x}$

   $x = (150 \text{ mg} \times 5 \text{ mL}) \div 500 \text{ mg} = 1.5 \text{ mL}$

   b. How many mLs are needed for one day?

   $1.5 \text{ mL} \times 4 = 6 \text{ mL}$

4. How many 300 mg doses can be made from 5400 mg?

   $5400 \text{ mg} \div 300 \text{ mg} = 18 \text{ doses}$

5. Amoxicillin is available in 250 mg/5 mL concentration. A patient needs 375 mg four times a day for 14 days.

   a. How many mLs will be needed for one dose?

   $$\frac{250 \text{ mg}}{5 \text{ mL}} = \frac{375 \text{ mg}}{x}$$

   $x = (375 \text{ mg} \times 5 \text{ mL}) \div 250 \text{ mg} = 7.5 \text{ mL}$

   b. How many mLs will be needed for the entire 14 days?

   7.5 mL × 4 = 30 mL × 14 days = 420 mL

6. The pharmacy has an order for gentamicin 170 mg. The concentration of the stock solution is 40 mg/mL. How much is needed for this dose?

   $$\frac{40 \text{ mg}}{1 \text{ mL}} = \frac{170 \text{ mg}}{x}$$

   $x = (170 \text{ mg} \times 1 \text{ mL}) \div 40 \text{ mg} = 4.25 \text{ mL}$

7. Dexamethasone elixir is available in 4 mg/5 mL concentration. The patient needs a 10 mg dose daily for 7 days.

   a. How many mLs is a 10 mg dose?

   $$\frac{4 \text{ mg}}{5 \text{ mL}} = \frac{10 \text{ mg}}{x}$$

   $x = (10 \text{ mg} \times 5 \text{ mL}) \div 4 \text{ mg} = 12.5 \text{ mg}$

   b. How much is needed for the full 7 days?

   12.5 mg × 7 days = 87.5 mL

8. Codeine 40 mg is ordered. The stock vial is 60 mg/2 mL. How many mLs are needed for the dose?

   $$\frac{60 \text{ mg}}{2 \text{ mL}} = \frac{40 \text{ mg}}{x}$$

   $x = (40 \text{ mg} \times 2 \text{ mL}) \div 60 \text{ mg} = 1.33 \text{ mL}$

9. Ferrous sulfate comes in 220 mg/5 mL concentration. How many mgs are in 7.5 mL?

   $$\frac{220 \text{ mg}}{5 \text{ mL}} = \frac{x}{7.5 \text{ mL}}$$

   $x = (220 \text{ mg} \times 7.5 \text{ mL}) \div 5 \text{ mL} = 330 \text{ mg}$

10. Potassium chloride liquid is available in 20 mEq/15 mL concentration. The patient needs 50 mEq two times a day.

    a. How much will be used for one dose?

    $$\frac{20 \text{ mEq}}{15 \text{ mL}} = \frac{50 \text{ mEq}}{x}$$

    $x = (50 \text{ mEq} \times 15 \text{ mL}) \div 20 \text{ mEq} = 37.5 \text{ mL}$

    b. How much will be used daily?

    37.5 mL × 2 doses = 75 mL

CHAPTER 4

Chapter 4 Quiz

1. What is the specific gravity of a liquid with a volume of 15 mL and a mass of 30 g?

    $$sg = \frac{30\ g}{15\ mL} = 2.0$$

2. What is the specific gravity of an acid with a mass of 62 g and a volume of 40 mL?

    $$sg = \frac{62\ g}{40\ mL} = 1.55$$

3. What is the specific gravity of a solution with a volume of 120 mL and a mass of 60 g?

    $$sg = \frac{60\ g}{120\ mL} = 0.5$$

4. What is the specific gravity of 2 oz of glycerin with a mass of 78 g? (*Hint:* 1 oz = 30 mL)

    $$sg = \frac{78\ g}{60\ mL} = 1.3$$

5. What is the specific gravity of 1 L of phenol with a mass of 1450 g? (*Hint:* 1 L = 1000 mL)

    $$sg = \frac{1450\ g}{1000\ mL} = 1.45$$

6. Alcohol has a specific gravity of 0.81. What is the volume if the mass is 125 g?

    $$sg = \frac{m}{v}$$

    $$0.81 = \frac{125\ g}{x}$$

    $$0.81x = 125\ g$$

    $$x = \frac{125\ g}{0.81} = 154.321 = 154.32$$

7. What is the mass of mercury if the specific gravity is 13.6 and the volume is 50 mL?

    $$sg = \frac{m}{v}$$

    $$13.6 = \frac{x}{50\ mL}$$

    $$13.6 \times 50\ mL = x$$

    $$x = 680\ g$$

8. A bottle of cough syrup weighs 16 oz and has a volume of 240 mL. What is the specific gravity? (*Hint:* 1 oz = 30 g)

    $$sg = \frac{480\ g}{240\ mL} = 2.0$$

9. The mass of antacid liquid is 360 g with a specific gravity of 1.6. What is the volume?

$$sg = \frac{m}{v}$$
$$1.6 = \frac{360 \text{ g}}{x}$$
$$1.6x = 360 \text{ g}$$
$$x = \frac{360 \text{ g}}{1.6}$$
$$x = 225 \text{ mL}$$

10. The volume of a cleaning agent that has a specific gravity of 1.2 is 946 mL. What is the mass?

$$sg = \frac{m}{v}$$
$$1.2 = \frac{x}{946 \text{ mL}}$$
$$1.2 \times 946 \text{ mL} = x$$
$$x = 1135.20 \text{ g}$$

CHAPTER 5

Practice Problems 5.1

1. How much tobramycin powder should be added to 240 g of an ointment base to obtain 4% w/w?

$$4\% = \frac{4 \text{ g}}{100 \text{ g}} \text{ so, } \frac{4 \text{ g}}{100 \text{ g}} = \frac{x}{240 \text{ g}}$$
$$x = (4 \text{ g} \times 240 \text{ g}) \div 100 \text{ g} = 9.6 \text{ g}$$

2. What is the % v/v concentration of 50 mL phenol added to 750 mL sterile water?

$$\frac{50 \text{ mL}}{800 \text{ mL}} = x\%$$
$$x = 50 \text{ mL} \div 800 \text{ mL} = 0.0625 \times 100 = 6.25\%$$

Hint: Remember that the fraction is volume of drug over total (final) volume.

3. How many grams of clindamycin 3% ointment can be made from 500 g of clindamycin powder?

$$3\% = \frac{3 \text{ g}}{100 \text{ g}} \text{ so, } \frac{3 \text{ g}}{100 \text{ g}} = \frac{x}{500 \text{ g}}$$
$$x = (3 \text{ g} \times 500 \text{ g}) \div 100 \text{ g} = 15 \text{ g}$$

4. What is the % w/v of a solution with a concentration of 50 mg/mL?

$$\frac{50 \text{ mg}}{1 \text{ mL}} = \frac{0.05 \text{ g}}{1 \text{ mL}} \text{ so, } \frac{0.05 \text{ g}}{1 \text{ mL}} = \frac{x}{100 \text{ mL}}$$

$x = (0.05 \text{ g} \times 100 \text{ mL}) \div 1 \text{ mL} = 5 \text{ g} = 5\%$

5. A stock acid has a concentration of 50% v/v. How many milliliters will be needed to make 240 mL of a 2% solution?

$$2\% = \frac{2 \text{ g}}{100 \text{ mL}} \text{ so, } \frac{2 \text{ g}}{100 \text{ mL}} = \frac{x}{240 \text{ mL}}$$

$x = (2 \text{ g} \times 240 \text{ mL}) \div 100 \text{ mL} = 4.8 \text{ g}$ acid total in 240 mL

$$50\% = \frac{50 \text{ mL}}{100 \text{ mL}} = \frac{4.8 \text{ g}}{x}$$

$x = (4.8 \text{ g} \times 100 \text{ mL}) \div 50 \text{ mL} = 9.6 \text{ mL}$

6. An IV containing dextrose has a concentration of 70% w/v. How many grams of dextrose are in 600 mL?

$$\frac{70 \text{ g}}{100 \text{ mL}} = \frac{x}{600 \text{ mL}}$$

$x = (70 \text{ g} \times 600 \text{ mL}) \div 100 \text{ mL} = 420 \text{ g}$

7. What is the percent strength of a promethazine syrup made from 50 g of promethazine powder in 480 mL?

$$\frac{50 \text{ g}}{480 \text{ mL}} = \frac{x}{100 \text{ mL}}$$

$x = (50 \text{ g} \times 100 \text{ mL}) \div 480 \text{ mL} = 10.4 \text{ g} = 10.4\%$

8. What is the % w/v of a ferrous sulfate solution of 300 mg/5 mL?

$$\frac{300 \text{ mg}}{5 \text{ mL}} = \frac{0.3 \text{ g}}{5 \text{ mL}} = \frac{x}{100 \text{ mL}}$$

$x = (0.3 \text{ g} \times 100 \text{ mL}) \div 5 \text{ mL} = 6 \text{ g} = 6\%$

9. How many grams of dextrose are needed to make 3000 mL of a 5% w/v solution?

$$5\% = \frac{5 \text{ g}}{100 \text{ mL}} = \frac{x}{3000 \text{ mL}}$$

$x = (5 \text{ g} \times 3000 \text{ mL}) \div 100 \text{ mL} = 150 \text{ g}$

10. How many grams of talc should be used to prepare 500 g of an 8% w/w gel?

$$8\% = \frac{8 \text{ g}}{100 \text{ g}} = \frac{x}{500 \text{ g}}$$

$x = (8 \text{ g} \times 500 \text{ g}) \div 100 \text{ g} = 40 \text{ g}$

Practice Problems 5.2

1. Convert 0.25% to ratio strength.

$$0.25\% = \frac{0.25}{100} = \frac{1}{x}$$
$$x = (1 \times 100) \div 0.25 = 400 = 1{:}400$$

2. Convert 1:200 to percent strength.

$$\frac{1}{200} = \frac{x\%}{100\%}$$
$$x = (1 \times 100) \div 200$$
$$x = \frac{100}{200} = 0.5\%$$

3. Convert 1:2500 to percent strength.

$$\frac{1}{2500} = \frac{x\%}{100\%}$$
$$x = (1 \times 100) \div 2500 = \frac{100}{2500} = 0.04\%$$

4. Convert 0.0125% to ratio strength.

$$\frac{0.0125}{100} = \frac{1}{x}$$
$$x = (1 \times 100) \div 0.0125 = 8000$$
$$x = \frac{100}{0.0125} = 1{:}8000$$

5. Convert 1:10,000 to mg/mL.

$$\frac{1\ g}{10{,}000\ mL} = \frac{1000\ mg}{10{,}000\ mL} = (1000\ mg \div 10{,}000\ mL) = 0.1\ mg/mL$$

6. Convert 4% to mg/mL.

$$4\% = \frac{4\ g}{100\ mL} = \frac{4000\ mg}{100\ mL} = 40\ mg/mL$$

7. A 30 mL vial of epinephrine 1:1000 contains how many milligrams of epinephrine?

$$\frac{1\ g}{1000\ mL} = \frac{1000\ mg}{1000\ mL} = \frac{x}{30\ mL}$$
$$x = (1000\ mg \times 30\ mL) \div 1000\ mL = 30\ mg$$

8. What is the ratio strength of a 4 mg/mL solution?

$$\frac{4 \text{ mg}}{1 \text{ mL}} = \frac{x}{100 \text{ mL}}$$

$x = (4 \text{ mg} \times 100 \text{ mg}) \div 1 \text{ mL} = 400 \text{ mg} = 0.4 \text{ g}$

$$\frac{0.4 \text{ g}}{100 \text{ mL}} = \frac{1}{x}$$

$x = (1 \times 100) \div 0.4 = 250$

$x = \frac{100 \text{ mL}}{0.4} = 1{:}250$

9. Midazolam is available in 5 mg/mL strength. What is its ratio strength?

$$\frac{5 \text{ mg}}{1 \text{ mL}} = \frac{x}{100 \text{ mL}}$$

$x = (5 \text{ mg} \times 100 \text{ mL}) \div 1 \text{ mL} = 500 \text{ mg} = 0.5 \text{ g}$

$$\frac{0.5}{100} = \frac{1}{x}$$

$x = (1 \times 100) \div 0.5 = 200$

$x = \frac{100}{0.5} = 1{:}200$

10. An anesthesiologist requests a solution with 3% cocaine and 1:4000 adrenaline for nasal application. How many milligrams of each solution will be needed for a 30 mL vial?

$$\text{Cocaine } 3\% = \frac{3 \text{ g}}{100 \text{ mL}} = \frac{x}{30 \text{ mL}}$$

$x = (3 \text{ g} \times 30 \text{ mL}) \div 100 \text{ mL} = 0.9 \text{ g} = 900 \text{ mg}$

$$\text{Adrenaline } 1{:}4000 = \frac{1 \text{ g}}{4000 \text{ mL}} = \left(\frac{1000 \text{ mg}}{4000 \text{ mL}} = \frac{x}{30 \text{ mL}} \right)$$

$x = (1000 \text{ mg} \times 30 \text{ mL}) \div 4000 \text{ mL} = 7.5 \text{ mg}$

Chapter 5 Quiz

Determine the total milligrams in each of the following medications.

1. Clindamycin 2% w/w cream 15 g tube

$$2\% = \frac{2 \text{ g}}{100 \text{ g}} = \left(\frac{2000 \text{ mg}}{100 \text{ g}} = \frac{x}{15 \text{ g}} \right)$$

$x = (2000 \text{ mg} \times 15 \text{ g}) \div 100 \text{ g} = 300 \text{ mg}$

2. Gentamicin 0.1% w/w ointment 20 g tube

$$0.1\% = \frac{0.1 \text{ g}}{100 \text{ g}} = \left(\frac{100 \text{ mg}}{100 \text{ g}} = \frac{x}{20 \text{ g}} \right)$$

$x = (100 \text{ mg} \times 20 \text{ g}) \div 100 \text{ g} = 20 \text{ mg}$

3. Metronidazole 0.5% w/w cream 45 g tube

$$0.5\% = \frac{0.5 \text{ g}}{100 \text{ g}} = \left(\frac{500 \text{ mg}}{100 \text{ g}} = \frac{x}{45 \text{ g}} \right)$$

$x = (500 \text{ mg} \times 45 \text{ g}) \div 100 \text{ g} = 225 \text{ mg}$

4. Dextrose 50% w/v solution 750 mL

$$50\% = \frac{50 \text{ g}}{100 \text{ mL}} = \left(\frac{50,000 \text{ mg}}{100 \text{ mL}} = \frac{x}{750 \text{ mL}} \right)$$

$x = (50,000 \text{ mg} \times 750 \text{ mL}) \div 100 \text{ mL} = 375,000 \text{ mg}$

5. Iodine 14% w/v solution 120 mL

$$14\% = \frac{14 \text{ g}}{100 \text{ mL}} = \left(\frac{14,000 \text{ mg}}{100 \text{ mL}} = \frac{x}{120 \text{ mL}} \right)$$

$x = (14,000 \text{ mg} \times 120 \text{ mL}) \div 100 \text{ mL} = 16,800 \text{ mg}$

6. Zinc oxide 3% w/w ointment 454 g

$$3\% = \frac{3 \text{ g}}{100 \text{ g}} = \left(\frac{3000 \text{ mg}}{100 \text{ g}} = \frac{x}{454 \text{ g}} \right)$$

$x = (3000 \text{ mg} \times 454 \text{ g}) \div 100 \text{ g} = 13,620 \text{ mg}$

7. Sodium chloride 23.4% w/v solution 60 mL

$$23.4\% = \frac{23.4 \text{ g}}{100 \text{ mL}} = \left(\frac{23,400 \text{ mg}}{100 \text{ mL}} = \frac{x}{60 \text{ mL}} \right)$$

$x = (23,400 \text{ mg} \times 60 \text{ mL}) \div 100 \text{ mL} = 14,040 \text{ mg}$

Determine the total milliliters of each medication in solution.

1. Alcohol 12% v/v 240 mL

$$12\% = \frac{12 \text{ mL}}{100 \text{ mL}} = \frac{x}{240 \text{ mL}}$$

$x = (12 \text{ mL} \times 240 \text{ mL}) \div 100 \text{ mL} = 28.80 \text{ mL}$

2. Albuterol 0.04% v/v inhalation solution 300 mL

$$0.04\% = \frac{0.04 \text{ mL}}{100 \text{ mL}} = \frac{x}{300 \text{ mL}}$$

$x = (0.04 \text{ mL} \times 300 \text{ mL}) \div 100 \text{ mL} = 0.12 \text{ mL}$

3. Thymol 0.05% solution in 250 mL

$$0.05\% = \left(\frac{0.05 \text{ mL}}{100 \text{ mL}} = \frac{x}{250 \text{ mL}} \right)$$

$x = (0.05 \text{ mL} \times 250 \text{ mL}) \div 100 \text{ mL} = 0.125 \text{ mL}$

Calculate the percent strength.

1. Dextrose 70 g in 500 mL

$$\frac{70 \text{ g}}{500 \text{ mL}} = \frac{x}{100 \text{ mL}}$$

$x = (70 \text{ g} \times 100 \text{ mL}) \div 500 \text{ mL} = 14 \text{ g} = 14\%$

2. Sodium chloride 12 g in 400 mL

$$\frac{12 \text{ g}}{400 \text{ mL}} = \frac{x}{100 \text{ mL}}$$

$x = (12 \text{ g} \times 100 \text{ mL}) \div 400 \text{ mL} = 3 \text{ g} = 3\%$

3. Lidocaine ointment 30 g in 480 g

$$\frac{30 \text{ g}}{480 \text{ g}} = \frac{x}{100 \text{ g}}$$

$x = (30 \text{ g} \times 100 \text{ g}) \div 480 \text{ g} = 6.25 \text{ g} = 6.25\%$

4. Nitroglycerin ointment 1.2 g in 60 g

$$\frac{1.2 \text{ g}}{60 \text{ g}} = \frac{x}{100 \text{ g}}$$

$x = (1.2 \text{ g} \times 100 \text{ g}) \div 60 \text{ g} = 2 \text{ g} = 2\%$

5. Amikacin 500 mg/mL

$$\frac{500 \text{ mg}}{1 \text{ mL}} = \left(\frac{0.5 \text{ g}}{1 \text{ mL}} = \frac{x}{100 \text{ mL}} \right)$$

$x = 0.5 \text{ g} \times 100 \text{ mL} = 50 \text{ g} = 50\%$

6. Promethazine 50 mg/mL

$$\frac{50 \text{ mg}}{1 \text{ mL}} = \left(\frac{0.05 \text{ g}}{1 \text{ mL}} = \frac{x}{100 \text{ mL}} \right)$$

$x = 0.05 \text{ g} \times 100 \text{ mL} = 5 \text{ g} = 5\%$

7. 1:250

$$\frac{1}{250} = \frac{x\%}{100\%}$$

$x = (100 \times 1) \div 250 = 0.4\%$

8. 1:400

$$\frac{1}{400} = \frac{x\%}{100\%}$$

$x = (100 \times 1) \div 400 = 0.25\%$

9. 1:1000

$$\frac{1}{1000} = \frac{x\%}{100\%}$$

$x = (100 \times 1) \div 1000 = 0.1\%$

10. Powder X 150 g dissolved in 1000 mL

$$\frac{150 \text{ g}}{1000 \text{ mL}} = \frac{x}{100 \text{ mL}}$$

$$x = (150 \text{ g} \times 100 \text{ mL}) \div 1000 \text{ mL} = 15 \text{ g} = 15\%$$

11. Erythromycin 6 g in 120 g

$$\frac{6 \text{ g}}{120 \text{ g}} = \frac{x}{100 \text{ g}}$$

$$x = (6 \text{ g} \times 100 \text{ g}) \div 120 \text{ g} = 5 \text{ g} = 5\%$$

12. Tobramycin 3 mg/mL

$$\frac{3 \text{ mg}}{1 \text{ mL}} = \left(\frac{0.003 \text{ g}}{1 \text{ mL}} = \frac{x}{100 \text{ mL}} \right)$$

$$x = (0.003 \text{ g} \times 100 \text{ mL}) \div 1 \text{ mL} = 0.3 \text{ g} = 0.3\%$$

Calculate the ratio strength.

1. Betamethasone 0.01%

$$\frac{0.01}{100} = \frac{1}{x}$$
$$x = (100 \times 1) \div 0.01 = 10,000$$

$$x = \frac{100}{0.01} = 10,000 = 1:10,000$$

2. Midazolam 5 mg/mL

$$\frac{5 \text{ mg}}{1 \text{ mL}} = \left(\frac{0.005 \text{ g}}{1 \text{ mL}} = \frac{x}{100 \text{ mL}} \right)$$

$$x = 0.005 \text{ g} \times 100 \text{ mL} = 0.5 \text{ g} = 0.5\%$$

$$\frac{0.5}{100} = \frac{1}{x}$$
$$x = (100 \times 1) \div 0.5 = 200$$

$$x = \frac{5 \text{ mg}}{1 \text{ mL}} = 1:200$$

3. 2.5%

$$2.5\% = \frac{2.5}{100} = \frac{1}{x}$$
$$x = (100 \times 1) \div 2.5$$
$$x = 2.5\% = 1:40$$

4. 0.8%

$$0.8\% = \frac{0.8}{100} = \frac{1}{x}$$
$$x = (100 \times 1) \div 0.8 = 125$$
$$x = 0.8\% = 1:125$$

5. 1 mg/0.5 mL

$$\frac{1 \text{ mg}}{0.5 \text{ mL}} = \left(\frac{0.001 \text{ g}}{0.5 \text{ mL}} = \frac{x}{100 \text{ mL}} \right)$$

$x = (0.001 \text{ g} \times 100 \text{ mL}) \div 0.5 \text{ mL} = 0.2 \text{ g} = 0.2\%$

$$\frac{0.2}{100} = \frac{1}{x}$$

$x = (100 \times 1) \div 0.2 = 500$

$x = \dfrac{1 \text{ mg}}{0.5 \text{ mL}} = 1{:}500$

6. Timolol 0.02%

$$\frac{0.02}{100} = \frac{1}{x}$$

$x = (100 \times 1) \div 0.02 = 5000$

$x = 0.02\% = 1{:}5000$

Solve the following problems.

1. Dissolve 2400 mg of tobramycin powder in 120 mL. What is the %w/v?

$$\frac{2400 \text{ mg}}{120 \text{ mL}} = \left(\frac{2.4 \text{ g}}{120 \text{ mL}} = \frac{x}{100 \text{ mL}} \right)$$

$x = (2.4 \text{ g} \times 100 \text{ mL}) \div 120 \text{ mL} = 2 \text{ g} = 2\% \text{ w/v}$

2. Combine 50 g of zinc oxide with 400 g of an ointment base. What is the %w/w?

$$\frac{50 \text{ g}}{450 \text{ g}} = \frac{x}{100 \text{ g}}$$

$x = (50 \text{ g} \times 100 \text{ g}) \div 450 \text{ g} = 11.1 \text{ g} = 11.1\% \text{ w/w}$

3. Add 150 mL water to 7.5 g of amoxicillin powder. What is the percent strength?

$$\frac{7.5 \text{ g}}{150 \text{ mL}} = \frac{x}{100 \text{ mL}}$$

$x = (7.5 \text{ g} \times 100 \text{ mL}) \div 150 \text{ mL} = 5 \text{ g} = 5\%$

4. How many milliliters of phenol and diluent must be combined to create a solution of 12% v/v 1000 mL?

$\text{Phenol} = \dfrac{12 \text{ mL}}{100 \text{ mL}} = \dfrac{x}{1000 \text{ mL}}$

$x = (12 \text{ mL} \times 1000 \text{ mL}) \div 100 \text{ mL} = 120 \text{ mL}$

Diluent $= 1000 \text{ mL} - 120 \text{ mL} = 880 \text{ mL}$

5. How much silver nitrate is needed to make 4 L of a 0.5% solution?

$0.5\% = \left(\dfrac{0.5 \text{ g}}{100 \text{ mL}} = \dfrac{x}{4000 \text{ mL}} \right)$

$x = (0.5 \text{ g} \times 4000 \text{ mL}) \div 100 \text{ mL} = 20 \text{ g}$

CHAPTER 6

Practice Problems 6.1

1. Sodium acetate 5% solution 100 mL is diluted to a volume of 1000 mL. What is the new percent strength?

$$5\% = \frac{5\ g}{100\ mL}$$

$$\frac{5\ g}{1000\ mL} = \frac{x}{100\ mL}$$

$$x = (5\ g \times 1000\ mL) \div 100\ mL = 0.5\ g = 50\%$$

2. A solution of 1:400 concentration 250 mL is diluted to 1000 mL. What is the new ratio strength?

$$1{:}400 = \frac{1}{400} = 0.0025 \times 100 = 0.25\% = \frac{0.25\ g}{100\ mL} = \frac{x}{250\ mL}$$

$$x = 0.625\ g\ in\ 250\ mL$$

$$\frac{0.625\ g}{1000\ mL} = \frac{x}{100\ mL} = 0.0625\ g = \frac{0.0625\%}{100\%} = \frac{1}{x}$$

$$x = \frac{100}{0.625} = 1600 = 1{:}1600$$

3. Niconozole 3% 60 g ointment is combined with 120 g of ointment base. What is the new percent strength?

$$3\% = \frac{3\ g}{100\ g} = \frac{x}{60\ g}$$

$$x = (3\ g \times 60\ g) \div 100\ g = 1.8\ g\ niconozole$$

$$\frac{1.8\ g}{180\ g} = \frac{x}{100\ g}$$

$$x = (1.8\ g \times 100\ g) \div 180\ g = 1\%$$

$$x = (180\ g = 60\ g + 120\ g)$$

4. How many milliliters of 4.2% sodium bicarbonate solution can be made from 100 mL of 8.4% concentration?

$$(C1 \times Q1 = C2 \times Q2)$$

$$8.4\% \times 100\ mL = 4.2\% \times x\ mL$$

$$x = 840 \div 4.2 = 200\ mL$$

(proportion equation)

$$8.4\% = \frac{8.4\ g}{100\ mL} = 8.4\ g\ 100\ mL\ stock\ solution$$

$$4.2\% = \frac{4.2\ g}{100\ mL} = \frac{8.4\ g}{x}$$

$$x = (8.4\ g \times 100\ mL) \div 4.2\ g = 200\ mL$$

5. How many grams of betamethasone 0.1% cream can be made from 60 g of a 1% concentration?

(proportion equation)

$$1\% = \frac{1\text{ g}}{100\text{ g}} = \frac{x}{60\text{ g}}$$

$x = (60\text{ g} \times 1\text{ g}) \div 100\text{ g} = 0.6\text{ g}$ in 60 g stock ointment

$$0.1\% = \frac{0.1\text{ g}}{100\text{ g}} = \frac{0.6\text{ g}}{x}$$

$x = (0.6\text{ g} \times 100\text{ g}) \div 0.1\text{ g} = 600\text{ g}$

$(C1 \times Q1 = C2 \times Q2)$

$1\% \times 60\text{ g} = 0.1\% \times x$

$x = (1 \times 60) \div 0.1 = 600\text{ g}$

6. How many milliliters of a 10% potassium solution are needed to make 180 mL of a 10mg/mL concentration solution?

$$\frac{10\text{ mg}}{\text{mL}} = \frac{1000\text{ mg}}{100\text{ mL}} = \frac{1\text{ g}}{100\text{ mL}} = 1\%$$

$$\frac{1\text{ g}}{100\text{ mL}} = \frac{x}{180\text{ mL}}$$

$x = (1\text{ g} \times 180\text{ mL}) \div 100\text{ mL} = 1.8\text{ g needed}$

$$\frac{1.8\text{ g}}{x} = \frac{10\text{ g}}{100\text{ mL}}$$

$x = (1.8\text{ g} \times 100\text{ mL}) \div 10\text{ g} = 18\text{ mL}$

7. How much diphenhydramine 2% ointment and how much ointment base are needed to make a 1 lb jar of diphenhydramine 0.5% ointment? (*Hint:* 1 lb = 454 g)

$$\frac{0.5\text{ g}}{100\text{ g}} = \frac{x}{454\text{ g}}$$

$x = (0.5\text{ g} \times 454\text{ g}) \div 100\text{ g} = 2.27\text{ g}$ diphenhydramine in 1 lb

$$2\% = \frac{2\text{ g}}{100\text{ g}} = \frac{2.27\text{ g}}{x}$$

$x = (2.27\text{ g} \times 100\text{ g}) \div 2\text{ g} = 113.5\text{ g}$ diphenhydramine ointment needed

$454\text{ g} - 113.5\text{ g}$ (diphenhydramine) $= 340.5\text{ g}$ ointment base

8. How many milliliters of 2% lidocaine are needed to make a 250 mL solution containing 0.4 mg/mL?

$$\frac{0.4\text{ mg}}{\text{mL}} = \frac{40\text{ mg}}{100\text{ mL}} = \frac{0.04\text{ g}}{100\text{ mL}} = 0.04\%, \quad \frac{0.04\text{ g}}{100\text{ mL}} = \frac{x}{250\text{ mL}}$$

$x = (0.04\text{ g} \times 250\text{ mL}) \div 100\text{ mL} = 0.1\text{ g needed}$

$$\frac{0.1\text{ g}}{x} = \frac{2\text{ g}}{100\text{ mL}}$$

$x = (0.1\text{ g} \times 100\text{ mL}) \div 2\text{ g} = 5\text{ mL}$

9. Hydrocortisone 5% ointment 120 g is added to enough ointment base to make a total volume of 1 lb. What is the new percent strength of hydrocortisone ointment? (*Hint:* 1 lb = 454 g)

$$\frac{5\text{ g}}{100\text{ g}} = \frac{x}{120\text{ g}}$$

$$x = (5\text{ g} \times 120\text{ g}) \div 100\text{ g} = 6\text{ g hydrocortisone in 1 lb}$$

$$\frac{6\text{ g}}{454\text{ g}} = \frac{x}{100\text{ g}}$$

$$x = (6\text{ g} \times 100\text{ g}) \div 454\text{ g} = 1.32\%$$

10. Cefotaxime comes in 10 g/100 mL concentration. How much diluent must be added to make a concentration of 50 mg/mL?

$$\frac{10\text{ g}}{100\text{ mL}} = 10\%; \frac{50\text{ mg}}{\text{mL}} = \frac{0.05\text{ g}}{\text{mL}} = \frac{5\text{ g}}{100\text{ mL}} = 5\% \text{ solution desired}$$

$$10\% \times 100\text{ mL} = 5\% \times x$$

$$x = (1000 \div 5) = 200\text{ mL } (C1 \times Q1 = C2 \times Q2)$$

Practice Problems 6.2

1. What is the percent strength of a solution containing 400 mL of 50% dextrose, 200 mL of 30% dextrose, and 400 mL of 10% dextrose?

$$50\% = \frac{50\text{ g}}{100\text{ mL}} = \frac{x}{400\text{ mL}}$$

$$x = 200\text{ g}$$

$$30\% = \frac{30\text{ g}}{100\text{ mL}} = \frac{x}{200\text{ mL}}$$

$$x = 60\text{ g}$$

$$10\% = \frac{10\text{ g}}{100\text{ mL}} = \frac{x}{400\text{ mL}}$$

$$x = 40\text{ g}$$

200 g in 400 mL

60 g in 200 mL

$$\frac{40\text{ g in 400 mL}}{300\text{ g in 1000 mL}} = \frac{300\text{ g}}{1000\text{ mL}} = \frac{x}{100\text{ mL}}$$

$$x = 30\text{ g} = 30\%$$

2. How many total grams of aminosyn are in a solution containing 200 mL of 8.5%, 150 mL of 5%, and 50 mL of 10% concentrations?

$8.5\% = \dfrac{8.5\text{ g}}{100\text{ mL}} = \dfrac{x}{200\text{ mL}}$

$x = 17$ g

$5\% = \dfrac{5\text{ g}}{100\text{ mL}} = \dfrac{x}{150\text{ mL}}$

$x = 7.5$ g

$10\% = \dfrac{10\text{ g}}{100\text{ mL}} = \dfrac{x}{50\text{ mL}}$

$x = 5$ g

17 g in 200 mL

7.5 g in 150 mL

$\dfrac{5\text{ g in 50 mL}}{29.5\text{ g in 400 mL}} = \dfrac{29.5\text{ g}}{400\text{ mL}} = \dfrac{x}{100\text{ mL}}$

$x = 7.375 = 7.38\%$

3. A 70% solution and 20% solution are combined to make a 30% solution. What is the ratio?

$\begin{pmatrix} 70 & \rightarrow & 10 \\ & 30 & \\ 20 & \rightarrow & 40 \end{pmatrix} = 10{:}40 = 1{:}4$ (1 part 70%, 4 parts 20%)

4. Dextrose 40% 1000 mL is needed for a patient. The pharmacy only stocks 20% and 50% solutions. How much of each is needed to make the solution?

$\begin{pmatrix} 50 & \rightarrow & 20 \\ & 40 & \\ 20 & \rightarrow & 10 \end{pmatrix} = 20{:}10 = 2{:}1$ ratio (2 parts 50%, 1 part 20%)

2 parts + 1 part = 3 parts total, 1000 mL/3 parts = 333.3 mL per part

1 part 20% = 333 mL, 2 parts 50% = 333.3 × 2 = 667 mL

5. How much 23.4% sodium chloride should be added to 300 mL of sterile water to make a 3% sodium chloride solution? (*Hint:* Remove decimal for calculation—move it to the right one place in both values.)

$\begin{pmatrix} 234\ (23.4\%) & \rightarrow & 30 \\ & 30\ (3\%) & \\ 0\ (\text{water}) & \rightarrow & 204 \end{pmatrix} = 30{:}204 = 5{:}34$ ratio

5 parts + 34 parts = 39 parts total, 300 mL/39 parts = 7.69 mL per part

5 parts 23.4% = 5 × 7.69 mL = 38.5 mL, 34 parts 0% (water)
$\qquad\qquad = 34 \times 7.69 = 261.5$ mL

6. What is the new percent strength when the following zinc oxide ointments are combined?

(Zinc 10% 60 g, zinc 6% 120 g, zinc 3% 120 g, zinc 5% 150 g)

$$10\% = \frac{10\text{ g}}{100\text{ g}} = \frac{x}{60\text{ g}}$$

$x = 6$ g

$$6\% = \frac{6\text{ g}}{100\text{ g}} = \frac{x}{120\text{ g}}$$

$x = 7.2$ g

$$3\% = \frac{3\text{ g}}{100\text{ g}} = \frac{x}{120\text{ g}}$$

$x = 3.6$ g

$$5\% = \frac{5\text{ g}}{100\text{ g}} = \frac{x}{150\text{ g}}$$

$x = 7.5$ g

6 g in 60 g

7.2 g in 120 g

3.6 g in 120 g

$\underline{7.5 \text{ g in } 150 \text{ g}}$

$$24.3 \text{ g in } 450 \text{ g} = \frac{24.3\text{ g}}{450\text{ g}} = \frac{x}{100\text{ g}}$$

$x = 5.4$ g $= 5.4\%$

7. How much 95% dextrose and how much 40% dextrose are needed to obtain a 70% concentration?

$$\begin{pmatrix} 95 & \rightarrow & 30 \\ & 70 & \\ 40 & \rightarrow & 25 \end{pmatrix} = 30{:}25 = 6{:}5 \text{ ratio (6 parts 95\% to 5 parts 40\%)}$$

8. Potassium chloride 20% 500 mL is ordered. The stock solutions available are 40% and 10%. How much of each is needed to make this solution?

$$\begin{pmatrix} 40 & \rightarrow & 10 \\ & 20 & \\ 10 & \rightarrow & 20 \end{pmatrix} = 10{:}20 = 1{:}2 \text{ ratio}$$

2 parts + 1 part = 3 parts total, 500 mL/3 parts = 166.6 mL per part

1 part 40% = 167 mL, 2 parts 10% = 166.6 × 2 = 333 mL

9. How much of each, 20% lidocaine and 30% lidocaine, are needed to make 500 mL of a 28% concentration?

$$\begin{pmatrix} 30 & \rightarrow & 8 \\ & 28 & \\ 20 & \rightarrow & 2 \end{pmatrix} = 8{:}2 = 4{:}1 \text{ ratio}$$

4 parts + 1 part = 5 parts total, 500 mL/5 = 100 mL per part

1 part 20% = 100 mL, 4 parts 30% = 100 mL × 4 = 400 mL

10. Housekeeping needs 1500 mL of a 34% cleansing solution. The stock solutions available are 18% and 42%. How much of each will be used?

$$\begin{pmatrix} 42 & \rightarrow & 16 \\ & 34 & \\ 18 & \rightarrow & 8 \end{pmatrix} = 16:8 = 2:1 \text{ ratio}$$

2 parts + 1 part = 3 parts total, 1500 mL/3 = 500 mL per part

1 part 18% = 500 mL, 2 parts 42% = 500 mL × 2 = 1000 mL

Chapter 6 Quiz

1. What is the final concentration (% strength) when you mix 800 g of hydrocortisone 5% cream and 1200 g of hydrocortisone 10% cream?

$$5\% = \frac{5 \text{ g}}{100 \text{ g}} = \frac{x}{800 \text{ g}}$$

$x = 40$ g

$$10\% = \frac{10 \text{ g}}{100 \text{ g}} = \frac{x}{1200 \text{ g}}$$

$x = 120$ g

40 g + 120 g = 160 g hydrocortisone

800 g + 1200 g = 2000 g volume (mass)

$$\frac{160 \text{ g}}{2000 \text{ g}} = \frac{x}{100 \text{ g}}$$

$x = 8$ g $= 8\%$

2. How many grams of dexamethasone 1% ointment can be made from 120 g of dexamethasone 5% ointment?

$5\% \times 120 \text{ g} = 1\% \times x$

$x = 600 \div 1 = 600$ g

3. How many milliliters of gentamicin 0.25% ophthalmic solution can be made from a 5 mL stock bottle of gentamicin 2.5% ophthalmic solution?

$2.5\% \times 5 \text{ mL} = 0.25\% \times x$

$x = 12.5 \div 0.25 = 50$ mL

4. What is the percent strength of epinephrine 1:5000, 1 mL diluted to a volume of 10 mL?

$$\frac{1 \text{ g (1000 mg)}}{5000 \text{ mL}} = \frac{x}{1 \text{ mL}}$$

$x = 0.2$ mg; $\dfrac{0.2 \text{ mg}}{10 \text{ mL}} = \dfrac{2 \text{ mg}}{100 \text{ mL}} = \dfrac{0.002 \text{ g}}{100 \text{ mL}} = 0.002\%$

5. A 50% alcohol solution is needed. How many milliliters of sterile water need to be added to 2500 mL of an 83% alcohol solution?

$$\begin{pmatrix} 83 & \rightarrow & 50 \\ & 50 & \\ 0 & \rightarrow & 33 \end{pmatrix} = 50{:}33 \text{ ratio}$$

50 parts = 83% (2500 mL) so 2500 mL ÷ 50 parts = 50 mL per part

33 parts = 0% (water) so 33 × 50 mL = 1650 mL

6. Terconazole 8% cream 30 g is diluted to 120 g with cream base. What is the new percent strength?

$$8\% = \frac{8 \text{ g}}{100 \text{ g}} = \frac{x}{30 \text{ g}}$$

$$x = 2.4 \text{ g}$$

$$\frac{2.4 \text{ g}}{120 \text{ g}} = \frac{x}{100 \text{ g}}$$

$$x = 2 \text{ g} = 2\%$$

7. An IV calls for a 500 mL–5% lipid solution. The stock solution available is 20%. How many milliliters of 20% lipids and how many milliliters of sterile water are needed for this IV?

$$\begin{pmatrix} 20 & \rightarrow & 5 \\ & 5 & \\ 0 & \rightarrow & 15 \end{pmatrix} = 5{:}15 = 1{:}3 \text{ ratio}$$

1 part + 3 parts = 4 parts total, 500 mL/4 parts = 125 mL per part

1 part 20% = 125 mL, 3 parts 0% = 3 × 125 mL = 375 mL

8. A patient needs 50 mL of a 5% dextrose solution. How many milliliters of 70% dextrose and how many milliliters of water will be needed to make this solution?

$$\begin{pmatrix} 70 & \rightarrow & 5 \\ & 5 & \\ 0 & \rightarrow & 65 \end{pmatrix} = 5{:}65 = 1{:}13 \text{ ratio}$$

1 part + 13 parts = 14 parts total, 50 mL/14 parts = 3.57 mL per part

1 part 70% = 3.6 mL, 13 parts of 0% = 13 × 3.57 = 46.4 mL

9. A stock bottle of calcium gluconate has concentration of 10 mg/mL. The prescription calls for 10 mL of a 4 mg/mL concentration. How many milliliters of calcium gluconate and how many milliliters of water are needed to fill this prescription?

$$\frac{4 \text{ mg}}{1 \text{ mL}} \times 10 \text{ mL} = 40 \text{ mg calcium gluconate needed for final concentration}$$

$$\frac{10 \text{ mg}}{1 \text{ mL}} = \frac{40 \text{ mg}}{x}$$

$x = 4$ mL calcium gluconate

10 mL − 4 mL = 6 mL water

10. Folic acid 50 mcg/mL, 30 mL is ordered. The stock vial is 5 mg/mL. How many milliliters of folic acid and how many milliliters of sterile water must be combined to fill this order?

$$\frac{50 \text{ mcg}}{\text{mL}} \times 30 \text{ mL} = 1500 \text{ mcg} = 1.5 \text{ mg} \text{ folic acid needed for final concentration}$$

$$\frac{5 \text{ mg}}{\text{mL}} = \frac{1.5 \text{ mg}}{x}$$

$x = 0.3$ mL folic acid

30 mL − 0.3 mL = 29.7 mL water

11. An IV of dextrose 12.5% 500 mL is ordered. The pharmacy only stocks D10%W and D20%W. How many milliliters of each will be needed?

$$\begin{pmatrix} 20 & \rightarrow & 2.5 \\ & 12.5 & \\ 10 & \rightarrow & 7.5 \end{pmatrix} = 2.5{:}7.5 = 1{:}3 \text{ ratio}$$

1 part + 3 parts = 4 parts total, 500 mL/4 parts = 125 mL

1 part 20% = 125 mL, 3 parts 10% = 125 mL × 3 = 375 mL

12. Dextrose 8% 400 mL is ordered. Make this solution from D20% and sterile water. How many milliliters of each solution will be needed?

$$\begin{pmatrix} 20 & \rightarrow & 8 \\ & 8 & \\ 0 & \rightarrow & 12 \end{pmatrix} = 8{:}12 = 2{:}3 \text{ ratio}$$

2 parts + 3 parts = 5 parts total, 400 mL ÷ 5 = 80 mL per part

2 parts 20% = 80 × 2 = 160 mL, 3 parts 0% = 3 × 80 = 240 mL

13. Sodium chloride 0.45% 500 mL is ordered. Make this solution from 23.4% sodium chloride and sterile water. How many milliliters of each will be needed? (*Hint:* Eliminate decimals for an easier calculation.)

$$\begin{pmatrix} 2340(23.4) & \rightarrow & 45 \\ & 45 & \\ 0 & \rightarrow & 2295 \end{pmatrix} 45{:}2295 = 1{:}51 \text{ ratio}$$

1 part + 51 parts = 52 parts total, 500 mL/52 parts = 9.6 mL per part

1 part 23.4% = 9.6 mL, 51 parts 0% = 9.6 × 51 = 490.4 mL

14. Triamcinolone cream 3% 60 g is needed. The stock available is a 10% cream and a 1% cream. How many grams of each will be used?

$$\begin{pmatrix} 10 & \rightarrow & 2 \\ & 3 & \\ 1 & \rightarrow & 7 \end{pmatrix} = 2{:}7 \text{ ratio}$$

2 parts + 7 parts = 9 parts total, 60 g ÷ 9 parts = 6.67 g per part

2 parts 10% = 6.67 × 2 = 13.3 g, 7 parts 1% = 6.67 × 7 = 46.7 g

15. Isoproterenol 1:400 20 mL is combined with isoproterenol 1:150 80 mL. What is the new concentration in ratio strength? In percent strength?

$$\frac{1\text{ g}}{400\text{ mL}} = \frac{x}{20\text{ mL}}$$

$$x = 0.05\text{ g}$$

$$\frac{1\text{ g}}{150\text{ mL}} = \frac{x}{80\text{ mL}}$$

$$x = 0.53\text{ g}$$

$$\frac{0.05\text{ g} + 0.53\text{ g}}{20\text{ mL} + 80\text{ mL}} = \frac{0.58\text{ g}}{100\text{ mL}} = 0.58\%$$

$$\frac{0.58\%}{100\%} = \frac{1}{x}$$

$$x = 172.4 = 1{:}172$$

16. Metronidazole cream 2% 30 g is mixed with metronidazole cream 8% 30 g. What is the new percent strength?

$$2\% = \frac{2\text{ g}}{100\text{ g}} = \frac{x}{30\text{ g}}$$

$$x = 0.6\text{ g}$$

$$8\% = \frac{8\text{ g}}{100\text{ g}} = \frac{x}{30\text{ g}}$$

$$x = 2.4\text{ g}$$

$$\frac{0.6\text{ g} + 2.4\text{ g}}{30\text{ g} + 30\text{ g}} = \frac{3\text{ g}}{60\text{ g}} = \frac{x}{100\text{ g}}$$

$$x = 5\text{ g} = 5\%$$

17. Mix together dextrose 15% 1000 mL, dextrose 3% 500 mL, dextrose 70% 300 mL, and dextrose 40% 200 mL. What is the new percent concentration?

$$15\% = \frac{15\text{ g}}{100\text{ mL}} = \frac{x}{1000\text{ mL}}$$

$$x = 150\text{ g}$$

$$3\% = \frac{3\text{ g}}{100\text{ mL}} = \frac{x}{500\text{ mL}}$$

$$x = 15\text{ g}$$

$$70\% = \frac{70\text{ g}}{100\text{ mL}} = \frac{x}{300\text{ mL}}$$

$$x = 210\text{ g}$$

$$40\% = \frac{40\text{ g}}{100\text{ mL}} = \frac{x}{200\text{ mL}}$$

$$x = 80\text{ g}$$

150 g in 1000 mL
 15 g in 500 mL
210 g in 300 mL
 80 g in 200 mL
_____
455 g in 2000 mL $= \dfrac{455\ g}{2000\ mL} = \dfrac{x}{100\ mL}$

$x = 22.75\ g = 22.75\%$

18. Mix together alcohol 50% 100 mL, alcohol 95% 100 mL, and alcohol 70% 100 mL. What is the new percent concentration?

$50\% = \dfrac{50\ g}{100\ mL} = 50\ g; 95\% = \dfrac{95\ g}{100\ mL} = 95\ g; 70\% = \dfrac{70\ g}{100\ mL} = 70\ g$

50 g in 100 mL
95 g in 100 mL
70 g in 100 mL
_____
215 g in 300 mL $= \dfrac{215\ g}{300\ mL} = \dfrac{x}{100\ mL}$

$x = 71.67\ g = 71.7\%$

19. Combine betamethasone 0.1% ointment 60 g, betamethasone 1% ointment 60 g, and betamethasone 3% ointment 120 g. What is the new percent strength?

$0.1\% = \dfrac{0.1\ g}{100\ g} = \dfrac{x}{60\ g}$

$x = 0.06\ g$

$1\% = \dfrac{1\ g}{100\ g} = \dfrac{x}{60\ g}$

$x = 0.6\ g$

$3\% = \dfrac{3\ g}{100\ g} = \dfrac{x}{120\ g}$

$x = 3.6\ g$

0.06 g in 60 g
0.6 g in 60 g
3.6 g in 120 g
_____
4.26 g in 240 g $= \dfrac{4.26\ g}{240\ g} = \dfrac{x}{100\ g}$

$x = 1.775\ g = 1.78\%$

20. Prepare 4 L of 28% iodine solution. The stock solutions available are 16% and 32%. How many milliliters of each solution are needed?

$\begin{pmatrix} 32 & \to & 12 \\ & 28 & \\ 16 & \to & 4 \end{pmatrix} = 12{:}4 = 3{:}1$

3 parts + 1 part = 4 parts total, 4000 mL (4 L) ÷ 4 parts = 1000 mL per part

1 part 16% = 1000 mL, 3 parts 32% = 1000 mL × 3 = 3000 mL

CHAPTER 7

Practice Problems 7.1

Calculate the BSA.

1. Patient weighs 40 lbs and is 42 in. tall.

$$\sqrt{\frac{42 \text{ in.} \times 40 \text{ lbs}}{3131}} = \sqrt{0.5366} = 0.73 \text{ m}^2$$

2. Patient weighs 220 lbs and is 72 in. tall.

$$\sqrt{\frac{72 \text{ in.} \times 220 \text{ lbs}}{3131}} = \sqrt{5.0591} = 2.25 \text{ m}^2$$

3. Patient weighs 80 kg and is 175 cm tall.

$$\sqrt{\frac{175 \text{ cm} \times 80 \text{ kg}}{3600}} = \sqrt{3.8889} = 1.97 \text{ m}^2$$

4. Patient weighs 2 kg and is 41 cm tall.

$$\sqrt{\frac{41 \text{ cm} \times 2 \text{ kg}}{3600}} = \sqrt{0.0228} = 0.15 \text{ m}^2$$

Calculate the following doses.

5. Amikacin 5 mg/kg/dose and patient weighs 80 kg.

   5 mg × 80 kg = 400 mg dose

6. Amoxicillin 10 mg/kg/dose and patient weighs 33 lbs.

   33 lbs ÷ 2.2 kg = 15 kg
   15 kg × 10 mg = 150 mg dose

7. Ranitidine 2.5 mg/kg/dose and patient weighs 176 lbs.

   176 lbs ÷ 2.2 kg = 80 kg
   80 kg × 2.5 mg = 200 mg dose

8. Ticarcillin 200 mg/kg/day and patient weighs 25 kg.

   200 mg × 25 kg = 5000 mg dose

9. A patient weighing 55 lbs has an order for clindamycin every 8 hr. Clindamycin is dosed at 15 mg/kg/day. How much is each dose?

   55 lbs ÷ 2.2 kg = 25 kg
   25 kg × 15 mg = 375 mg per dose per day
   375 mg ÷ 3 = 125 mg per dose per 8 hr

Calculate the following doses using Young's Rule and Clark's Rule.

10. Ibuprofen is ordered for a 5-year-old child weighing 40 lbs. The adult dose is 600 mg.

Young's Rule: $\dfrac{5 \text{ yrs} \times 600 \text{ mg}}{5 \text{ yrs} + 12} = \dfrac{3000}{17} = 176.5 \text{ mg}$

Clark's Rule: $\dfrac{40 \text{ lbs} \times 600 \text{ mg}}{150} = 160 \text{ mg}$

11. Metronidazole is ordered for an 8-year-old child weighing 65 lbs. The adult dose is 500 mg.

Young's Rule: $\dfrac{8 \text{ yrs} \times 500 \text{ mg}}{8 \text{ yrs} + 12} = \dfrac{4000}{20} = 200 \text{ mg}$

Clark's Rule: $\dfrac{65 \text{ lbs} \times 500 \text{ mg}}{150} = 216.67 \text{ mg} = 217 \text{ mg}$

12. Diphenhydramine is ordered for a 2-year-old child weighing 20 lbs. The adult dose is 50 mg.

Young's Rule: $\dfrac{2 \text{ yrs} \times 50 \text{ mg}}{2 \text{ yrs} + 12} = \dfrac{100}{14} = 7.14 \text{ mg}$

Clark's Rule: $\dfrac{20 \text{ lbs} \times 50 \text{ mg}}{150} = 6.67 \text{ mg}$

13. Erythromycin is ordered for a 6-year-old child weighing 50 lbs. The adult dose is 1 g (1000 mg).

Young's Rule: $\dfrac{6 \text{ yrs} \times 1000 \text{ mg}}{6 \text{ yrs} + 12} = \dfrac{6000}{18} = 333.33 \text{ mg}$

Clark's Rule: $\dfrac{50 \text{ lbs} \times 1000 \text{ mg}}{150} = 333.33 \text{ mg}$

14. Metoclopramide is ordered for an 11-year-old child weighing 80 lbs. The adult dose is 10 mg.

Young's Rule: $\dfrac{11 \text{ yrs} \times 10 \text{ mg}}{11 \text{ yrs} + 12} = \dfrac{110}{23} = 4.78 \text{ mg}$

Clark's Rule: $\dfrac{80 \text{ lbs} \times 10 \text{ mg}}{150} = 5.33 \text{ mg}$

Practice Problems 7.2

Calculate the creatinine clearance.

1. Patient is a 65-year-old male and weighs 175 lbs. The serum creatinine is 1.9 mg/dL.

175 lbs ÷ 2.2 kg = 79.55 kg

$\text{CrCl} = \dfrac{(140 - 65 \text{ yrs}) \times 79.55 \text{ kg}}{72 \times 1.9 \text{ mg/dL}} = \dfrac{5966.25}{136.8} = 43.61 \text{ mL/min}$

2. Patient is a 42-year-old female and weighs 140 lbs. The serum creatinine is 1.2 mg/dL.

   140 lbs ÷ 2.2 kg = 63.64 kg

   $$CrCl = 0.85 \times \frac{(140 - 42 \text{ yrs}) \times 63.64 \text{ kg}}{72 \times 1.2 \text{ mg/dL}} = 0.85 \times \frac{6236.72}{86.4} = 61.36 \text{ mL/min}$$

3. Patient is an 84-year-old male and weighs 160 lbs. The serum creatinine is 2.1 mg/dL.

   160 lbs ÷ 2.2 kg = 72.73 kg

   $$CrCl = \frac{(140 - 84 \text{ yrs}) \times 72.73 \text{ kg}}{72 \times 2.1 \text{ mg/dL}} = \frac{4072.88}{151.2} = 26.94 \text{ mL/min}$$

4. Patient is a 75-year-old female and weighs 155 lbs. The serum creatinine is 1.8 mg/dL.

   155 lbs ÷ 2.2 kg = 70.45 kg

   $$CrCl = 0.85 \times \frac{(140 - 75 \text{ yrs}) \times 70.45 \text{ kg}}{72 \times 1.8 \text{ mg/dL}} = 0.85 \times \frac{4579.25}{129.6} = 30.03 \text{ mL/min}$$

5. Patient is a 90-year-old female and weighs 110 lbs. The serum creatinine is 2.0 mg/dL.

   110 lbs ÷ 2.2 kg = 50 kg

   $$CrCl = 0.85 \times \frac{(140 - 90 \text{ yrs}) \times 50 \text{ kg}}{72 \times 2.0 \text{ mg/dL}} = 0.85 \times \frac{2500}{144} = 14.76 \text{ mL/min}$$

Calculate the dose based on BSA and CrCl.

   Cyclophosphamide 500 mg/m²
   Reduce dose by 10% CrCl < 35 mL/min
   Reduce dose by 25% CrCl < 20 mL/min

6. Patient is a 75-year-old male, weighs 165 lbs, and is 67 in. tall with serum creatinine 1.8 mg/dL.

   165 lbs ÷ 2.2 kg = 75 kg

   $$BSA = \sqrt{\frac{67 \text{ in.} \times 165 \text{ lbs}}{3131}} = \sqrt{3.5308} = 1.88 \text{ m}^2$$

   $$CrCl = \frac{(140 - 75 \text{ yrs}) \times 75 \text{ kg}}{72 \times 1.8 \text{ mg/dL}} = \frac{4875}{129.6} = 37.61 \text{ mL/min}$$

   500 mg × 1.88 m² = 940 mg dose

7. Patient is a 62-year-old female, weighs 121 lbs, and is 65 in. tall with serum creatinine 1.7 mg/dL.

121 lbs ÷ 2.2 kg = 55 kg

$$BSA = \sqrt{\frac{65 \text{ in.} \times 121 \text{ lbs}}{3131}} = \sqrt{2.512} = 1.58 \text{ m}^2$$

$$CrCl = 0.85 \times \frac{(140 - 62 \text{ yrs}) \times 55 \text{ kg}}{72 \times 1.7 \text{ mg/dL}} = 0.85 \times \frac{4290}{122.4} = 29.79 \text{ mL/min}$$

500 mg × 1.58 m² = 790 mg dose − 10% reduction = 711 mg dose

Chapter 7 Quiz

Calculate the BSA. Remember to use the correct formula.

1. Patient is 60 in. tall and weighs 75 kg.

75 kg × 2.2 = 165 lbs

$$BSA = \sqrt{\frac{60 \text{ in.} \times 165 \text{ lbs}}{3131}} = \sqrt{3.1619} = 1.78 \text{ m}^2$$

2. Patient is 165 cm tall and weighs 70 kg.

$$BSA = \sqrt{\frac{165 \text{ cm} \times 70 \text{ kg}}{3600}} = \sqrt{3.2083} = 1.79 \text{ m}^2$$

3. Patient is 70 in. tall and weighs 200 lbs.

$$BSA = \sqrt{\frac{70 \text{ in.} \times 200 \text{ lbs}}{3131}} = \sqrt{4.4714} = 2.11 \text{ m}^2$$

4. Patient is 30 in. tall and weighs 32 lbs.

$$BSA = \sqrt{\frac{30 \text{ in.} \times 32 \text{ lbs}}{3131}} = \sqrt{0.3066} = 0.55 \text{ m}^2$$

5. Patient is 70 cm tall and weighs 20 lbs.

20 lbs ÷ 2.2 kg = 9.09 kg

$$BSA = \sqrt{\frac{70 \text{ cm} \times 9.09 \text{ kg}}{3600}} = \sqrt{0.1768} = 0.42 \text{ m}^2$$

Calculate the dose.

1. Medication is dosed at 12 mg/kg/day. The patient weighs 187 lbs.

187 lbs ÷ 2.2 kg = 85 kg
85 kg × 12 mg = 1020 mg daily

2. Cefazolin is ordered 75 mg/kg/day divided into three doses. The patient weighs 25 kg. How much is needed for one dose?

   75 mg × 25 kg = 1875 mg daily
   1875 mg ÷ 3 doses = 625 mg per dose

3. Gentamicin 1.75 mg/kg/dose. Patient weighs 132 lbs.

   132 lbs ÷ 2.2 kg = 60 kg
   60 kg × 1.75 mg = 105 mg dose

4. Hydrocortisone 0.5 mg/kg/dose. Patient weighs 60 kg.

   60 kg × 0.5 mg = 30 mg dose

5. Ibuprofen 20 mg/kg/day. Patient weighs 275 lbs.

   275 lbs ÷ 2.2 kg = 125 kg
   125 kg × 20 mg = 2500 mg daily

Calculate dose using BSA.

1. Paclitaxol is ordered at 135 mg/m². Patient weighs 132 lbs and is 66 in. tall.

   $$BSA = \sqrt{\frac{66 \text{ in.} \times 132 \text{ lbs}}{3131}} = \sqrt{2.7825} = 1.67 \text{ m}^2$$
   135 mg × 1.67 m² = 225.45 mg dose

2. Vincristine is ordered at 2 mg/m². Patient weighs 55 kg and is 167 cm tall.

   $$BSA = \sqrt{\frac{167 \text{ cm} \times 55 \text{ kg}}{3600}} = \sqrt{2.5514} = 1.60 \text{ m}^2$$
   (2 mg × 1.60 m² = 3.2 mg dose

   (*Note:* Vincristine has a maximum dose of 2 mg, so this would be reduced to 2 mg.)

3. Amikacin is ordered at 100 mg/m². Patient weighs 22 lbs and is 26 in. tall.

   $$BSA = \sqrt{\frac{26 \text{ in.} \times 22 \text{ lbs}}{3131}} = \sqrt{0.1827} = 0.43 \text{ m}^2$$
   100 mg × 0.43 m² = 43 mg dose

4. Carboplatin is ordered at 150 mg/m². Patient weighs 220 lbs and is 72 in. tall.

   $$BSA = \sqrt{\frac{72 \text{ in.} \times 220 \text{ lbs}}{3131}} = \sqrt{5.0591} = 2.25 \text{ m}^2$$
   150 mg × 2.25 m² = 337.50 mg dose

5. Methotrexate is ordered at 25 mg/m². Patient weighs 165 lbs and is 69 in. tall.

   $$BSA = \sqrt{\frac{69 \text{ in.} \times 165 \text{ lbs}}{3131}} = \sqrt{3.6362} = 1.91 \text{ m}^2$$
   25 mg × 1.91 m² = 47.75 mg dose

Calculate creatinine clearance.

1. Patient weighs 82 kg and is a 70-year-old male. Serum creatinine is 1.9 mg/dL

$$CrCl = \frac{(140 - 70 \text{ yrs}) \times 82 \text{ kg}}{72 \times 1.9 \text{ mg/dL}} = \frac{5740}{136.8} = 41.96 \text{ mL/min}$$

2. Patient is a 65-year-old female who weighs 150 lbs. Serum creatinine is 1.8 mg/dL.

150 lbs ÷ 2.2 kg = 68.18 kg

$$CrCl = 0.85 \times \frac{(140 - 65 \text{ yrs}) \times 68.18 \text{ kg}}{72 \times 1.8 \text{ mg/dL}} = 0.85 \times \frac{5113.5}{129.6} = 33.54 \text{ mL/min}$$

3. Patient is a 45-year-old female who weighs 135 lbs. Serum creatinine is 1.6 mg/dL.

135 lbs ÷ 2.2 kg = 61.36 kg

$$CrCl = 0.85 \times \frac{(140 - 45 \text{ yrs}) \times 61.36 \text{ kg}}{72 \times 1.6 \text{ mg/dL}} = 0.85 \times \frac{5829.2}{115.2} = 43.01 \text{ mL/min}$$

4. Patient weighs 65 kg and is a 92-year-old male. Serum creatinine is 2.1 mg/dL.

$$CrCl = \frac{(140 - 92 \text{ yrs}) \times 65 \text{ kg}}{72 \times 2.1 \text{ mg/dL}} = \frac{3120}{151.2} = 20.63 \text{ mL/min}$$

5. Patient weighs 125 kg and is a 54-year-old male. Serum creatinine is 1.7 mg/dL.

$$CrCl = \frac{(140 - 54 \text{ yrs}) \times 125 \text{ kg}}{72 \times 1.7 \text{ mg/dL}} = \frac{10,750}{122.4} = 87.83 \text{ mL/min}$$

Calculate the dose. Use the information provided to determine which formula is needed.

1. A patient weighs 12 kg. Acetaminophen w/codeine is ordered at 0.5 mg/kg/dose.

12 kg × 0.5 mg = 6 mg dose

2. A patient has a BSA of 0.82 m². Gangcyclovir 250 mg/m² is ordered.

250 mg × 0.82 m² = 205 mg dose

3. Mitomycin 25 mg/m² is ordered. Patient weighs 185 lbs and is 71 in. tall.

$$BSA = \sqrt{\frac{71 \text{ in.} \times 185 \text{ lbs}}{3131}} = \sqrt{4.1951} = 2.05 \text{ m}^2$$

25 mg × 2.05 m² = 51.25 mg dose

4. Acyclovir 250 mg/m² is ordered. Patient weighs 22 lbs and is 30 in. tall.

$$BSA = \sqrt{\frac{30 \text{ in.} \times 22 \text{ lbs}}{3131}} = \sqrt{0.2108} = 0.46 \text{ m}^2$$

250 mg × 0.46 m² = 115 mg dose

5. Ampicillin 40 mg/kg/day is ordered. Patient weighs 12 kg and is 2 years old.

40 mg × 12 kg = 480 mg daily

6. Erythromycin 50 mg/kg/day is ordered. Patient weighs 132 lbs and is 20 years old.

   132 lbs ÷ 2.2 kg = 60 kg

   60 kg × 50 mg = 3000 mg daily

7. Child is 8 years old. The adult dose of medication is 750 mg.

   Young's Rule: $\dfrac{8 \text{ yrs} \times 750 \text{ mg}}{8 \text{ yrs} + 12} = \dfrac{6000}{20} = 300$ mg

8. Child is 32 lbs. The adult dose of medication is 150 mg.

   Clark's Rule: $\dfrac{32 \text{ lbs} \times 750 \text{ mg}}{150} = 160$ mg

9. Levothyroxine 5 mcg/kg is ordered. The patient weighs 95 kg.

   5 mcg × 95 kg = 475 mcg dose

10. Cisplatin 150 mg/m² is ordered. The patient is a 58-year-old male, weighs 209 lbs, and is 69 in. tall. The serum creatinine is 1.8 mg/dL. The physician ordered a 10% dose reduction.

    209 lbs ÷ 2.2 kg = 95 kg

    a. What is the BSA?

    $$\text{BSA} = \sqrt{\dfrac{69 \text{ in.} \times 209 \text{ lbs}}{3131}} = \sqrt{4.6059} = 2.15 \text{ m}^2$$

    b. What is the CrCl?

    $$\text{CrCl} = \dfrac{(140 - 58 \text{ yrs}) \times 95 \text{ kg}}{72 \times 1.8 \text{ mg/dL}} = \dfrac{7790}{129.6} = 60.11 \text{ mL/min}$$

    c. What is the calculated dose?

    150 mg × 2.15 m² = 322.5 mg dose

    d. What is the reduced dose?

    322.5 mg − 10% = 290.25 mg dose

CHAPTER 8

Practice Problems 8.1

1. A physician ordered 15 mEq of potassium chloride in NS 100 mL. How much potassium chloride will be added to the NS? Potassium chloride is available as 2 mEq/mL.

   $$\dfrac{15 \text{ mEq}}{x} = \dfrac{2 \text{ mEq}}{1 \text{ mL}}$$

   $x = 7.5$ mL

2. Potassium phosphate 60 mEq/1000 mL is ordered. The patient has 750 mL remaining in the current IV bag. How much should be added to this current IV bag? Potassium phosphate is available as 4.4 mEq/mL.

$$\frac{60 \text{ mEq}}{1000 \text{ mL}} = \frac{x}{750 \text{ mL}}$$

$$x = 45 \text{ mEq}$$

$$\frac{45 \text{ mEq}}{x} = \frac{4.4 \text{ mEq}}{1 \text{ mL}}$$

$$x = 10.23 \text{ mL}$$

3. An order for regular insulin calls for 12 units/100 mL. The patient has a 500 mL bag of NS currently hanging. How many units of insulin must be added? How many milliliters of insulin are needed for the dose? Insulin is available as 100 units/mL.

$$\frac{12 \text{ units}}{100 \text{ mL}} = \frac{x}{500 \text{ mL}}$$

$$x = 60 \text{ units}$$

$$\frac{60 \text{ units}}{x} = x\frac{100 \text{ units}}{1 \text{ mL}}$$

$$x = 0.6 \text{ mL}$$

4. Penicillin 5 million units in NS 100 mL every 4 hr are ordered. How many milliliters are needed for one dose? Penicillin is available as 500,000 units/mL.

$$\frac{5,000,000 \text{ units}}{x} = \frac{500,000 \text{ units}}{1 \text{ mL}}$$

$$x = 10 \text{ mL}$$

5. Heparin 25,000 units/250 mL is ordered. The patient has 200 mL remaining in the IV bag. How much heparin should be added to the patient's IV bag? The heparin available is 10,000 units/mL.

$$\frac{25,000 \text{ units}}{250 \text{ mL}} = \frac{x}{200 \text{ mL}}$$

$$x = 20,000 \text{ units}$$

$$\frac{20,000 \text{ units}}{x} = \frac{10,000 \text{ units}}{1 \text{ mL}}$$

$$x = 2 \text{ mL}$$

Practice Problems 8.2

1. A patient has an IV order for LR 1500 mL at 80 mL/hr. What is the rate in gtts/min if the nurse uses a 60 gtts/mL set?

$$\text{gtts/min} = \frac{(80 \text{ mL/1 hr}) \times 60 \text{ gtts/mL}}{60 \text{ min/hr}} = \frac{4800}{60} = 80 \text{ gtts/min}$$

2. An IV is running at 100 mL/hr. How many 1000 mL bags are needed for a 24-hr period?

$$\frac{1000\ mL}{100\ mL/hr} = 10\ hr;\ \ 24\ hr/10\ hr = 2.4\ bags = 3\ bags$$

3. What is the gtts/min rate for a 50 mL bag of cimetidine if it is to run over 30 min using a 20 gtts/mL tubing?

$$gtts/min = \frac{(50\ mL/0.5\ hr) \times 20\ gtts/mL}{60\ min/hr} = \frac{2000}{60} = 33.33\ gtts/min$$

4. Lidocaine 0.4% 500 mL is ordered to run at 30 gtts/min. How long will the bag last if a 15 gtts/mL tubing is used?

$$mL/min = \frac{30\ gtts}{min} \times \frac{1\ mL}{15\ gtts} = 2\ mL/min$$

$$mL/hr = \frac{2\ mL}{min} \times \frac{1\ hr}{60\ min} = 120\ mL/hr$$

$$500\ mL/120\ mL = 4.16 = 4\ hr$$

5. Dextrose 5% 1000 mL will last for 12 hr. What is the rate in mL/hr?

$$1000\ mL/12\ hr = 83.3 = 83\ mL/hr$$

6. TPN Order:

   Dextrose 20% 500 mL

   Amino acids 5% 500 mL

   KCl 60 mEq   *(stock = 2 mEq/mL)*

   NaCl 40 mEq   *(stock = 4 mEq/mL)*

   CaGluc 750 mg   *(stock = 1 g/10 mL)*

   KPhos 15 mEq   *(stock = 4.4 mEq/mL)*

   Insulin 16 units   *(stock = 100 units/mL)*

   Base solution volume = 1000 mL

   Run this IV over 8 hr

   a. How much is needed of each additive for this TPN?

   $$KCl\ \frac{60\ mEq}{x} = \frac{2\ mEq}{1\ mL}$$

   $$x = 30\ mL$$

   $$NaCl\ \frac{40\ mEq}{x} = \frac{4\ mEq}{1\ mL}$$

   $$x = 10\ mL$$

   $$CaGluc\ \frac{750\ mg}{x} = \frac{1000\ mg\ (1\ g)}{10\ mL}$$

   $$x = 7.5\ mL$$

   $$KPhos\ \frac{15\ mEq}{x} = \frac{4.4\ mEq}{mL}$$

   $$x = 3.4\ mL$$

$$\text{Insulin} = \frac{16 \text{ units}}{x} = \frac{100 \text{ units}}{1 \text{ mL}}$$

$$x = 0.16 \text{ mL}$$

b. What is the rate in mL/hr?

1000 mL/8 hr = 125 mL/hr

c. What is the rate in gtts/min for a 60 gtts/mL tubing?

$$\text{gtts/min} = \frac{(125 \text{ mL/1 hr}) \times 60 \text{ gtts/min}}{60 \text{ min/hr}} = \frac{7500}{60} = 125 \text{ gtts/min}$$

Chapter 8 Quiz

1. Heparin 20,000 units/mL is available. How many units are in 0.6 mL?

$$\frac{20,000 \text{ units}}{1 \text{ mL}} = \frac{x}{0.6 \text{ mL}}$$

$$x = 12,000 \text{ units}$$

2. Penicillin G 4.5 million units is ordered for a patient. The pharmacy stocks a 500,000 units/mL solution. How many milliliters are needed for this order?

$$\frac{4,500,000 \text{ units}}{x} = \frac{500,000 \text{ units}}{1 \text{ mL}}$$

$$x = 9 \text{ mL}$$

3. D5 $\frac{1}{2}$ NS 1000 mL w/40 mEq KCl is ordered. How much potassium is needed if the pharmacy carries a 2 mEq/mL concentration?

$$\frac{40 \text{ mEq}}{x} = \frac{2 \text{ mEq}}{\text{mL}}$$

$$x = 20 \text{ mL}$$

4. NaCl 60 mEq/1000 mL is ordered. The patient only has 800 mL remaining in the IV bag. How much NaCl must be added if the stock solution is 4 mEq/mL?

$$\frac{60 \text{ mEq}}{1000 \text{ mL}} = \frac{x}{800 \text{ mL}}$$

$$x = 48 \text{ mEq}$$

$$\frac{48 \text{ mEq}}{x} = \frac{4 \text{ mEq}}{\text{mL}}$$

$$x = 12 \text{ mL}$$

5. Vitamin E 400 units are ordered. The pharmacy stocks 1000 units/5 mL. How much is needed for this dose?

$$\frac{400 \text{ units}}{x} = \frac{1000 \text{ units}}{5 \text{ mL}}$$

$$x = 2 \text{ mL}$$

6. LR 1000 mL will run from 7 AM to 3 PM.

   a. What is the rate in mL/hr?

      7 AM–3 PM = 8 hr; 1000 mL/8 hr = 125 mL/hr

   b. How much is remaining after 5 hr?

      125 mL × 5 hr = 625 mL; 1000 mL − 625 mL = 375 mL

   c. What is the rate in gtts/min for a 15 gtts/mL tubing?

$$\text{gtts/min} = \frac{(125 \text{ mL/hr}) \times 15 \text{ gtts/mL}}{60 \text{ min/hr}} = \frac{1875}{60} = 31.25 \text{ gtts/min}$$

7. NS 500 mL runs for 24 hr. What is the rate in mL/hr?

   500 mL ÷ 24 hr = 20.8 mL = 21 mL/hr

8. TPN Order:

   Dextrose 70% 1000 mL

   Amino acids 8.5% 1000 mL

   Lipids 20% 500 mL

   NaCl 30 mEq/1000 mL   *(stock = 4 mEq/mL)*

   KCl 15 mEq/1000 mL   *(stock = 2 mEq/mL)*

   Cimetidine 150 mg/1000 mL   *(stock = 300 mg/2 mL)*

   Insulin 5 units/1000 mL   *(stock = 100 units/mL)*

   Base solution volume = 2500 mL

   Run over 24 hr

   a. How much of each additive is needed?

$$\text{NaCl} = \frac{30 \text{ mEq}}{1000 \text{ mL}} = \frac{x}{2500 \text{ mL}}$$

$x = 75 \text{ mEq}$

$$\frac{75 \text{ mEq}}{x} = \frac{4 \text{ mEq}}{\text{mL}}$$

$x = 18.75 \text{ mL}$

$$\text{KCl} = \frac{15 \text{ mEq}}{1000 \text{ mL}} = \frac{x}{2500 \text{ mL}}$$

$x = 37.5 \text{ mEq}$

$$\frac{37.5 \text{ mEq}}{x} = \frac{2 \text{ mEq}}{\text{mL}}$$

$x = 18.75 \text{ mL}$

$$\text{Cimetidine} \frac{150 \text{ mg}}{1000 \text{ mL}} = \frac{x}{2500 \text{ mL}}$$

$x = 375 \text{ mg}$

$$\frac{375 \text{ mg}}{x} = \frac{300 \text{ mg}}{2 \text{ mL}}$$

$x = 2.5 \text{ mL}$

Insulin $\dfrac{5 \text{ units}}{1000 \text{ mL}} = \dfrac{x}{2500 \text{ mL}}$

$x = 12.5$ units

$\dfrac{12.5 \text{ units}}{x} = \dfrac{100 \text{ units}}{\text{mL}}$

$x = 0.125$ mL

b. What is the rate in mL/hr?

2500 mL ÷ 24 hr = 104.16 mL/hr = 104 mL/hr

c. What is the rate in gtts/min for a 20 gtts/mL tubing?

$\text{gtts/min} = \dfrac{(104 \text{ mL/hr}) \times 20 \text{ gtts/mL}}{60 \text{ min/hr}} = \dfrac{2080}{60} = 34.7 \text{ gtts/min}$

9. Vancomycin 750 mg in NS 250 mL is run over 90 min. What is the gtts/min for a 20 gtts/mL tubing?

$\text{gtts/min} = \dfrac{(250 \text{ mL} \div 1.5 \text{ hr}) \times 20 \text{ gtts/mL}}{60 \text{ min/hr}} = \dfrac{3333.3}{60} = 55.5 \text{ gtts/min}$

10. How long will a 1000 mL bag of D5LR last if it is running at 40 gtts/min through a 20 gtts/mL tubing?

$\text{mL/min} \dfrac{40 \text{ gtts}}{\text{min}} \times \dfrac{1 \text{ mL}}{20 \text{ gtts}} = 2 \text{ mL/min}$

$\text{mL/hr} \dfrac{2 \text{ mL}}{\text{min}} \times \dfrac{60 \text{ min}}{1 \text{ hr}} = 120 \text{ mL/hr}$

1000 mL ÷ 120 mL = 8.3 hr

CHAPTER 9

Practice Problems 9.1

1. The annual purchases for Pharmacy A totals $750,000. The average inventory is $192,000. What is the turnover rate?

   Turnover = $750,000 ÷ $192,000 = 3.9 turns

2. A prescription sells for $56. The medication cost is $22 and dispensing costs are $13. What is the gross profit? What is the net profit?

   Gross profit = $56 − $22 = $34
   Net profit = $56 − $22 − $13 = $21

3. A prescription sells for $110. The medication cost is $72 and dispensing costs are $22. What is the gross profit? What is the net profit?

   Gross profit = $110 − $72 = $38
   Net profit = $110 − $72 − $22 = $16

4. The pharmacy had annual purchases of $250,000. The average inventory is $100,000. What is the turnover rate?

   Turnover rate = $250,000 ÷ $100,000 = 2.5 turns

5. A prescription sells for $18. The medication cost is $4 and dispensing costs are $7.50. What is the gross profit? What is the net profit?

   Gross profit = $18 − $4 = $14
   Net profit = $18 − $4 − $7.50 = $6.50

Practice Problems 9.2

Calculate the selling price for the following prescriptions using the information provided.

Joe's Pharmacy
Markup percent = 18%
Dispensing fee = $6
Compounding fee = $60/hr
Senior discount = 10%

1. Furosemide 40 mg #100; Cost = $95/500 tablets

   $95.00/500 = 0.19 per tablet × 100 tablets = $19.00
   $19.00 + (0.18 × 19) + $6.00 = $19.00 + $3.42 + $6.00 = $28.42

2. Ranitidine 150 mg #30; Cost = $126/30 tablets

   $126.00 + (0.18 × 126) + $6.00 = $126.00 + $22.68 + $6.00 = $154.68

3. Digoxin 0.25 mg #90; Cost = $52/100 tablets, patient is a senior citizen

   $52.00/100 = 0.52 per tablet × 90 tablets = $46.80
   $46.80 + (0.18 × 46.80) + $6.00 = $46.80 + $8.42 + $6.00 = $61.22
   $61.22 − (0.1 × 61.22) = $61.22 − $6.12 = $55.10

4. | Camphor | 10 mL | $3.20 |
Glycerin	20 mL	$2.50
Zinc oxide	45 g	$12.00
Vitamin A ointment	45 g	$6.00

   Compounding time = 15 min

   $3.20 + $2.50 + $12.00 + $6.00 = $23.70
   $23.70 + (0.18 × 23.70) + $6.00 + compounding fee ($60.00/4) =
   $23.70 + $4.27 + $6.00 + $15.00 = $48.97

5. Promethazine syrup w/codeine 6 oz; Cost = $19.20/16 oz

   $19.20/16 oz = $1.20 per oz × 6 oz = $7.20
   $7.20 + (0.18 × 7.20) + $6.00 = $7.20 + $1.30 + $6.00 = $14.50

6. Amoxicillin 500 mg #28; Cost = $125/500 capsules

   $125/500 capsules = 0.25 per capsule × 28 capsules = $7

   $7.00 + (0.18 × 7) + $6.00 = $7.00 + $1.26 + $6.00 = $14.26

7. Clindamycin 300 mg #42; Cost = $108/60 capsules

   $108.00/60 capsules = $1.80 per capsule × 42 capsules = $75.60

   $75.60 + (0.18 × 75.60) + $6.00 = $75.60 + $13.61 + $6.00 = $95.21

8. Lanolin cream   30 g $4.80
   Vitamin E oil   10 mL $6.00
   Zinc oxide   60 g $12.20
   Talc powder   30 g $15.00
   Compounding time = 20 min, customer has a 5% coupon

   $4.80 + $6.00 + $12.20 + $15.00 = $38.00

   $38.00 + (0.18 × 38) + $6.00 + compounding fee ($60.00 ÷ 3)

     = $38.00 + $6.84 + $6.00 + $20.00 = $70.84 − (0.05 × 70.84)
     = $70.84 − $3.54 = $67.30

9. Regular insulin 10 mL #3 bottles; Cost = $22/bottle, patient is a senior citizen

   $22.00 × 3 bottles = $66.00 + (0.18 × 66) + $6.00 = $66.00 + $11.88
                      + $6.00 = $83.88

   $83.88 − (0.1 × 83.88) = $83.88 − $8.39 = $75.49

10. Lovastatin 20 mg #60; Cost = $216/120 tablets

    $216.00/120 = $1.80 per tablet × 60 tablets = $108.00

    $108.00 + (0.18 × 108) + $6.00 = $108.00 + $19.44 + $6.00 = $133.44

Practice Problems 9.3

1. Joe's Pharmacy receives a monthly capitation fee of $5000 from Insurance Company Z. This month he processed weekly claims of $1200, $700, $1400, and $1000. How much profit/loss did Joe record?

   $1200 + $700 + $1400 + $1000 = $4300

   $5000 − $4300 = $700 profit

2. Insurance A reimburses prescription claims for AWP − 7% + $4 per prescription. What is the total reimbursement for three prescriptions having a total AWP of $380?

   $380.00 − (0.07 × 380) + ($4.00 × 3) = $380.00 − $26.60 + $12.00 = $365.40

3. Which company has a better reimbursement rate? The AWP is $95.
   a. Insurance X = AWP − 4% + $2 per prescription

      $95.00 − (0.04 × 95) + $2.00 = $95.00 − $3.80 + $2.00 = $93.20

   b. Insurance Y = AWP − 10% + $4 per prescription

      $95.00 − (0.1 × 95) + $4.00 = $95.00 − $9.50 + $4.00 = $89.50

4. How much will Joe's Pharmacy receive for reimbursement on claims submitted to Insurance B that have a total AWP of $1800 for 40 prescriptions? They reimburse at AWP–6% + $2 per prescription.

$1800 − (0.06 × 1800) + ($2 × 40) = $1800 − $108 + $80 = 1772

5. Joe's Pharmacy received its monthly capitation fee from Insurance Y for $3500. The claims submitted each week were $500, $700, $1200, and $1400. How much was the profit/loss for the month?

$500 + $700 + $1200 + $1400 = 3800

$3500 − $3800 = ($300) loss$

Chapter 9 Quiz

1. The annual inventory for Pharmacy X is $700,000. Their average inventory is $175,000. What is their turnover rate?

Turnover = $700,000 ÷ $175,000 = 4 turns$

2. The turnover rate for Pharmacy Y is 5. Their average inventory is $72,000. What is their annual inventory?

$72,000 × 5 turns = $360,000 inventory$

3. Wholesaler T gives a 15% discount to pharmacies that pay their invoices within 15 days. Joe's Pharmacy always pays their invoices in time to receive the discount. They purchased a 100-capsule bottle of Indomethacin 50 mg. What is the cost of that bottle if the AWP is $185?

$185.00 − (0.15 × 185) = $185.00 − $27.75 = 157.25

4. Joe's Pharmacy dispensed acetaminophen w/codeine #3, 40 tablets. The selling price was $23.40. They cost of the medication was $16.20. What is the gross profit?

Gross profit = $23.40 − $16.20 = 7.20

5. Joe's Pharmacy dispensed Azithromycin 250 mg #14 tablets for $26.40. The cost of the medication was $14.20. The dispensing costs were $9.30. What is the net profit?

$26.40 − $14.20 − $9.30 = 2.90

For the following prescriptions, use the information below:

Markup = 12% for AWP less than $100
Markup = $5 for AWP $100 or more
Dispensing fee = $6 per prescription
Dispensing cost = $7.50
Compounding fee = $60 per hour
Senior citizen discount = 10%

6. Dispense #40 alprazolam 0.5 mg tablets; AWP = $48/100 tablets
   a. What is the selling price?

   $48.00/100 tablets = $0.48 per tablet × 40 tablets = $19.20 for 40 tablets$
   $19.20 + (0.12 × 19.20) + $6.00 = $19.20 + $2.30 + $6.00 = 27.50

   b. What is the gross profit?

     $27.50 − $19.20 = $8.30

   c. What is the net profit?

     $27.50 − $19.20 − $7.50 = $0.80

7. Dispense cefaclor 250 mg/5 mL 150 mL bottle; AWP = $102 per bottle
   a. What is the selling price?

     $102.00 + $5.00 + $6.00 = $113.00

   b. What is the gross profit?

     $113.00 − $102.00 = $11.00

   c. What is the net profit?

     $113.00 − $102.00 − $7.50 = $3.50

8. Dispense the following compounded prescription:

Betamethasone 1%	15 g	AWP = $15.40
Bacitracin ointment	15 g	AWP = $6.10
Aquaphor ointment	30 g	AWP = $4.50

   Compounding time = 10 min

   a. What is the selling price?

     $15.40 + $6.10 + $4.50 = $26.00

     $26.00 + (0.12 × 26) + $6.00 + compounding fee ($60.00/6) =

       $26.00 + $3.12 + $6.00 + $10.00 = $45.12

   b. What is the selling price for a senior citizen?

     $45.12 − (0.1 × 45.12) = $45.12 − $4.51 = $40.61

   c. What is the gross profit?

     $40.61 − $26.00 = $14.61

   d. What is the net profit?

     $40.61 − $26.00 − $7.50 = $7.11

9. Insurance Company A reimburses AWP − 7% + $2.50 per prescription. How much is Joe's reimbursement for:
   a. Prescription in Problem 6?

     $19.20 − (0.07 × $19.20) + $2.50 = $19.20 − $1.34 + $2.50 = $20.36

   b. Prescription in Problem 7?

     $102 − (0.07 × 102) + $2.50 = $102 − $7.14 + $2.50 = $97.36

   c. Prescription in Problem 8?

     $26.00 − (0.07 × 26) + $2.50 = $26.00 − $1.82 + $2.50 = $26.68

10. Insurance B reimburses AWP − 4% + $2 per prescription. How much is Joe's reimbursement for:

    a. Prescription in Problem 6?

       $19.20 − (0.04 × $19.20) + $2.00 = $19.20 − $0.77 + $2.00 = $20.43

    b. Prescription in Problem 7?

       $102.00 − (0.04 × 102) + $2.00 = $102.00 − $4.08 + $2.00 = $99.92

    c. Prescription in Problem 8?

       $26.00 − (0.04 × 26) + $2.00 = $26.00 − $1.04 + $2.00 = $26.96

Common Measures and Conversions

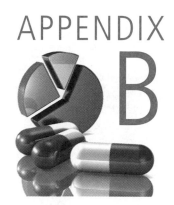

1 teaspoon (tsp)		5 mL	
1 tablespoon (tbsp)	3 teaspoons	15 mL	$\frac{1}{2}$ ounce (oz)
2 tablespoons	6 teaspoons	30 mL	1 oz
$\frac{1}{2}$ cup	8 tablespoons	120 mL	4 oz
1 cup	16 tablespoons	240 mL	8 oz
1 pint	2 cups	473–480 mL	16 oz
1 quart	2 pints	960–1000 mL	32 oz
1 gallon	4 quarts	3985–4000 mL	128 oz
2.2 pounds (lbs)	1 kg		
1 pound (lb)	454 g		
1 ounce (oz)	30 g		
4 ounces (oz)	120 g		
8 ounces (oz)	240 g		
1 inch (in.)	2.54 cm		
1 grain (gr)	60–65 mg		
1 gram (g)	1000 mg	1,000,000 mcg	
1 milligram (mg)		1000 mcg	
1 liter (L)	1000 mL	1,000,000 mcL	
1 milliliter (mL)	1 cubic centimeter (cc)		

Index

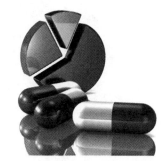